CLEAN EATING
COOKBOOK
for WEIGHT LOSS

28 Days

to Kick-Start

a Healthy

Lifestyle

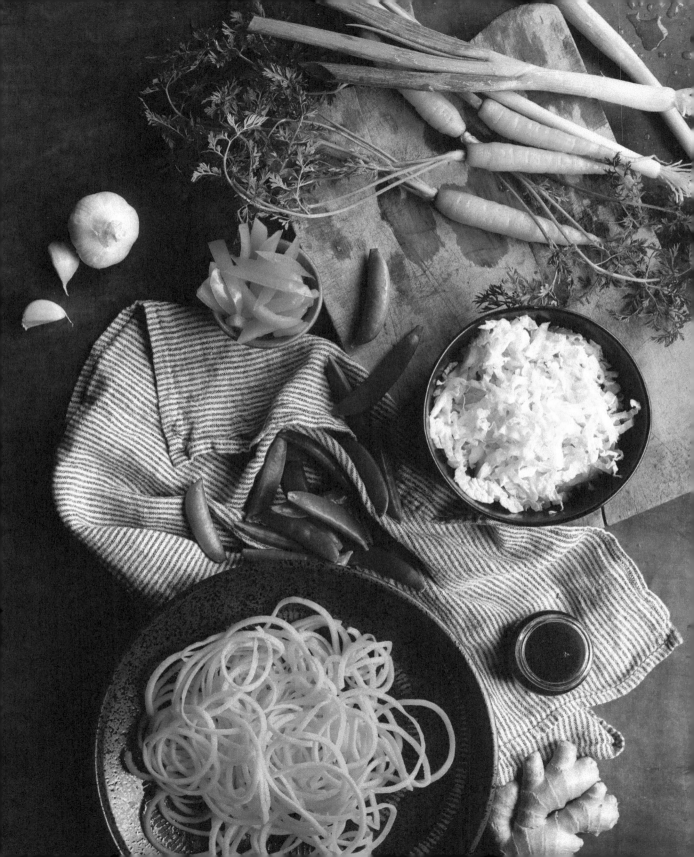

CLEAN EATING COOKBOOK
for WEIGHT LOSS

28 Days
to Kick-Start
a Healthy
Lifestyle

NIKKI BEHNKE

ROCKRIDGE
PRESS

Interior and Cover Designer: Amanda Kirk
Art Producer: Michael Hardgrove

Photography © 2019 Elysa Weitala. Food styling by Victoria Woollard.

Illustration © Charlie Layton.

Stock © Shutterstock/Anna Sedneva, iStock/Robyn Mac, Shutterstock/matin, p. 8; Shutterstock/sabyna75, p. 9; Shutterstock/Colorlife, Shutterstock/davooda, pp. 39, 46, 53, 60.

ISBN: Print 978-1-64611-472-6 | eBook 978-1-64611-473-3

R0

for

John,

Avery,

and

Keira

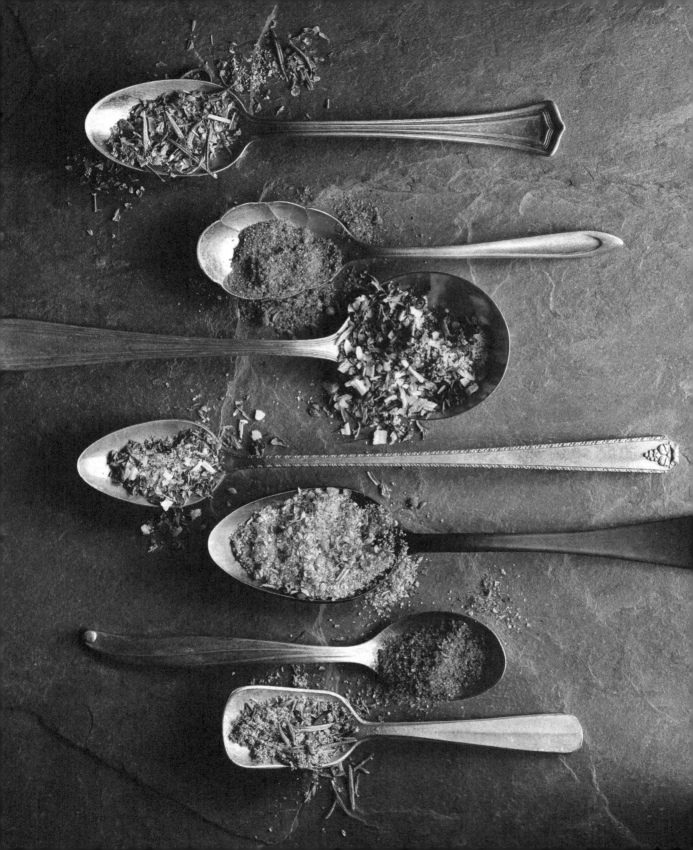

Contents

Clean eating

*a diet consisting mainly of whole,
real food coming from natural sources*

INTRODUCTION

My clean eating journey has been a labor of love, in more ways than one. As a teenager and young adult, I honestly never gave nutrition a second thought. Growing up, I ate what I wanted, never had a weight problem, and generally looked at food for entertainment or enjoyment purposes. Then I entered my late twenties and early thirties, had two babies, and was working a nine-to-five job. Not surprisingly, I became more sedentary and my energy level was lower than low, but I chalked it up to being a new parent with young kids. Most days, my lunch consisted of a sub sandwich, chips, and a Coke. Late-night snacks were also my jam, and breakfast was nonexistent. I gained a good amount of weight, began having regular digestive issues, and felt lethargic most of the time. It was a slow progression—but a progression, nonetheless—of unhealthy habits creeping into my daily life—with equally unhealthy results.

Over the years, I tried many popular diets and workout programs with some short-term success—usually followed by a crash-and-burn period. When I was suddenly faced with some significant career and life changes, I finally took pause to look seriously at my lifestyle and knew it was time to take action.

I experimented with several diet elimination programs, but quickly recognized that they were not a permanent weight-loss solution. It was around that time I was introduced to Michael Pollan's book *In Defense of Food* and discovered my general lack of awareness regarding the foods I was eating and feeding to my kids. It was an eye-opening process that would go on to awaken a passion in me. But it didn't happen overnight.

I slowly began to introduce clean eating practices into my family's routine by studying nutrition labels, eliminating processed junk, and planning and prepping my meals ahead of time. The extra weight began to fall off. I had more energy and was sleeping better than ever—something I had always struggled with. And then, things really evolved. I changed career paths, started a healthy recipe and wellness blog, and began studying to become a nutritional therapy practitioner. I haven't looked back.

Sometimes it takes a triggering moment or life event to make real change, but sometimes it's a gradual shift. Perhaps you've heard the buzz about clean eating and want to learn more. Maybe you're tired of feeling sluggish, or maybe you just want to lose weight. Whatever your reason for picking up this book, I hope you will welcome this opportunity to transform your health by embracing clean eating and exercise as a permanent lifestyle. And I look forward to guiding you!

PART ONE

The Clean Eating Plan

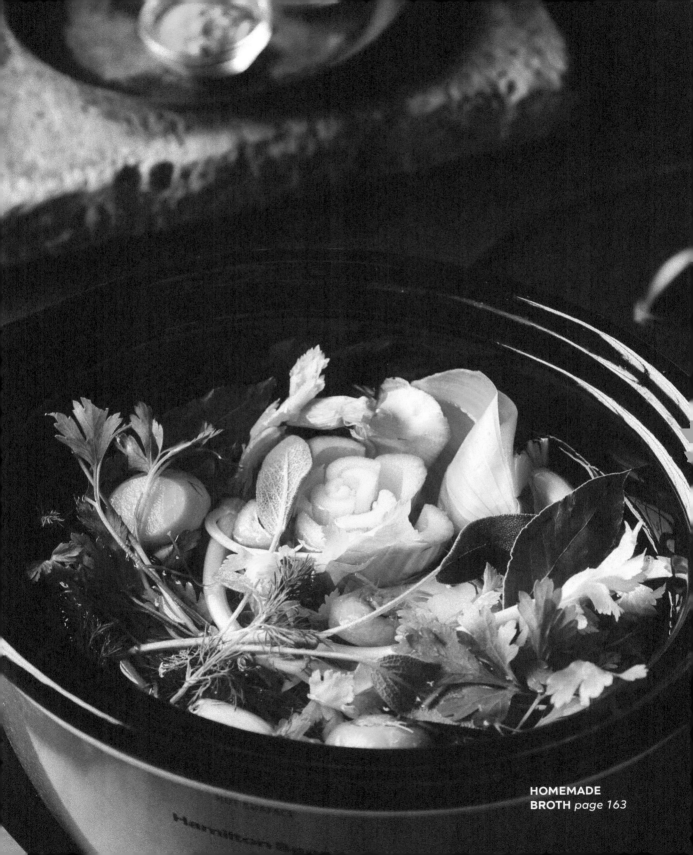

HOMEMADE
BROTH *page 163*

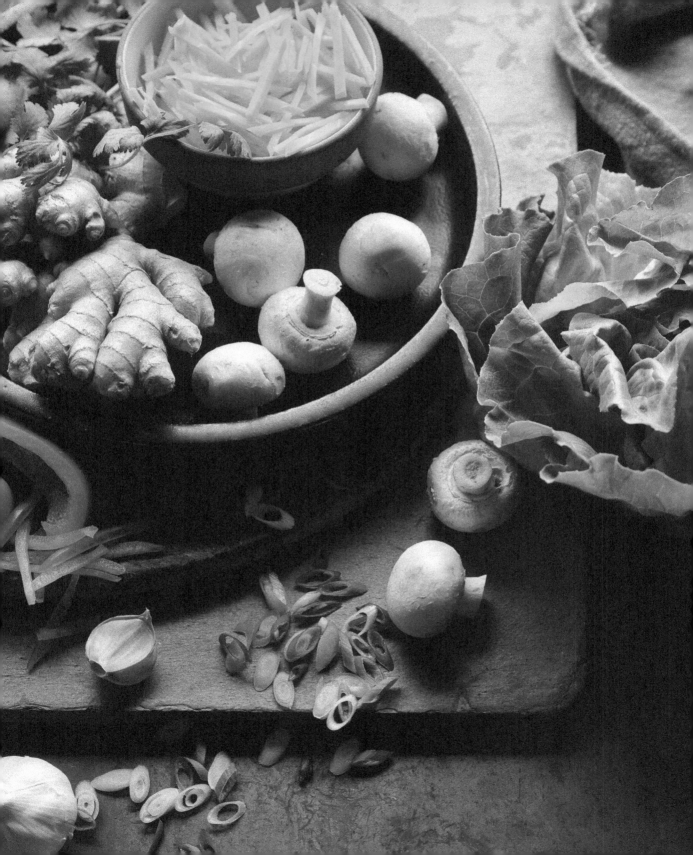

CHAPTER ONE

LOSING WEIGHT WITH CLEAN EATING

"Real food, real simple" is my motto for every recipe I publish on my website. My personal success has been rooted in this concept—get rid of the dieting mind-set, choose real food, plan ahead, and keep mealtime stress-free. You'll see that theme coming through in this book as well.

This 28-day plan is a holistic approach designed for anyone wanting to introduce healthy habits and shed some pounds in a realistic and lasting way. Together, we'll explore the concept of clean eating and how to implement it in your day-to-day life and, more importantly, how to adopt a manageable approach to eating and exercise for positive long-term results. Then we'll put that plan to work for you.

WHAT IS CLEAN EATING?

It's important to clarify right from the start that clean eating is not a diet, quick fix, or fad. Clean eating is a lifestyle. It's an approach to eating that is simple, straightforward, holistic in nature, and easy to sustain. The idea of clean eating has been around for decades but has recently increased in popularity. You've probably heard the term thrown around loosely, and while there are varying degrees and definitions out there, at its core, clean eating can be described as eating a diet consisting mainly of whole, real foods coming from natural sources. In simple terms, when we eat clean, it means we're consuming foods the way nature delivered them, or as close to it as possible.

A major cornerstone of clean eating is awareness—knowing what you're putting in your body, where it came from, and the impact it has on your health and mental well-being. I believe this self-education is the most important step we can take to improve our health.

Once we gain this awareness, we can use it to guide us in our food choices—both the food we put in our bodies and the food we bring into our homes. But rather than a structured diet full of rigid rules and restrictions, clean eating revolves around realistic and sustainable healthy food choices. Translation: Load up on vegetables, fruits, good-quality protein, healthy fats, and plant-based whole grains, while skipping the refined sugar, packaged convenience foods, and processed ingredients. Balance and moderation are key components as well, because life is meant to be enjoyed and occasional treats are never forbidden, but nutrient-dense food is the primary focus.

Health Benefits/Holistic Approach

Why adopt a clean eating lifestyle? Let's first discuss the alternative. Fast food, packaged snacks, soda, and sugar-laden treats have become far too common-place in society. Unfortunately, our bodies weren't designed to handle the highly processed fare that has become the standard American diet. In fact, processed foods currently account for nearly 60 percent of the American diet, or just under 1,200 calories per day. And while they often taste great (thanks to all the added sugar, sodium, and other additives), in excess these heavily pro-cessed convenience foods are doing serious damage. We are sending our bodies into overtime to try and process these food-like substances. When I look back on my days of eating fast food for lunch every day, it's no wonder I felt so lousy! Health concerns like obesity, autoimmune disease, and cancer are on the rise, and you can bet that the typical diet consisting of artificial ingredients and empty calories is not helping matters.

But there's plenty of good news, too. Research shows that consuming a nutrient-dense diet of whole foods over time works wonders for our physical well-being. A real-food approach to eating is proven to reduce inflammation, regulate blood sugar, heal autoimmune conditions, and lower the risk of disease.

That's not all. The benefits of a clean eating lifestyle go beyond just physical results. Besides encouraging natural weight loss and improved health, following a clean eating plan has been shown to improve mental clarity, increase mood and energy levels, and improve quality of sleep. Think of it this way: Food is fuel, and our bodies need the very best to function optimally, both physically *and* mentally.

The other benefit to eating a diet full of quality, nutritionally dense foods? It's totally sustainable over time—that is, you can get away with it forever, unlike many fad diets and weight-loss schemes. The key to maintaining weight loss and improved health overall is choosing a strategy that makes sense for the next four years, not just the next four weeks.

I love the clean eating approach because it is well-rounded and realistic for the whole family. If you're tired of trying to lose weight on a restrictive diet while your family members eat everything they want, this plan is for you. Adults and kids alike can get on board with the plan—and enjoy doing it!

10 Clean Eating Principles

Let's take a closer look at what it means to eat clean. The following guidelines are the pillars of a clean eating lifestyle. When you follow these 10 principles, you're on your way to a healthier, stronger, happier you!

1. **Eat whole foods.** Choose fruits, veggies, pure protein sources, and whole grains. The food should be nutrient-dense and as close to its natural state as possible. Ideally, it won't come from a factory or a box.

2. **Cut out processed food.** So much of what we consume is highly processed, food-like substances—sounds kind of gross when you think about
it that way, right? They lack nutrients for sure, but they often contain
harmful ingredients and additives. Common culprits to avoid are snack/
granola bars, soda, most breakfast cereals, salad dressings, chips, crackers,
and baked goods, even those labeled "all-natural" or with other misleading claims.

3. **Read nutrition labels.** If I could emphasize one thing, this would be it.
If it comes in a package, always check the nutrition label. Are there more
than five ingredients? Is sugar listed? Do you recognize the ingredients?
Awareness of what's in our food is the number one building block of
clean eating.

4. **Avoid refined sugar.** The bad news is that refined white sugar is toxic to
our bodies, promotes inflammation, and often leads to weight gain—and
it's highly addictive. The good news? This addiction goes away when it's
eliminated from the diet. We don't need refined sugar in our diets like we
need vitamins, minerals, and protein. Eliminate it whenever possible, and
use natural sweeteners like honey, pure maple syrup, and fruits instead.
Within a matter of weeks, you won't crave it like you did before. And as
your clean eating efforts become a way of life, you're likely to begin noticing that things with sugar just taste too sweet.

5. **Up your veggie intake.** Many of us were trained to build our meals
around meat and carbs, but in reality, they should be a pretty small portion of the plate. Start by filling half your plate with vegetables and build
from there.

6. **Include healthy fats.** Fat is not to be feared. By choosing the right fats
and including them with your meals, you'll feel full and satisfied longer.
Healthy fats include olives, avocado, coconut oil, nuts, seeds, fatty fish,
and eggs.

7. **Cook your own food.** To truly eat clean, you need to be in charge of what
goes into your food. The easiest way to do this is to cook your own meals at
home, where you control the ingredients. Restaurant meals are fine occasionally, but it's best to stick to homemade as much as possible.

8. **Drink LOTS of water.** Aim for at least half your body weight in ounces of water per day. Eliminate soda, fruit juices with added sugars (real and artificial), and other sweetened beverages—even some seemingly healthy flavored water drinks are nothing but empty calories.

9. **Choose carbs wisely.** Not all carbs are bad. Many diets promote eating zero carbs to lose weight, which is an effective strategy if weight loss is your only goal. But unless you intend to live your entire life without ever touching a carb again, you can plan to remain on the weight-loss roller coaster. The fact is, we need some carbohydrates in our diet for energy. Healthy carb options also contain high amounts of fiber, which aids in digestion. Complex carbs are best because they take longer to break down and digest, creating a more gradual impact on blood sugar—you can find complex carbs in fruit, whole grains, legumes, and starchy vegetables.

10. **Get moving.** Consistent exercise is an important part of overall wellness, no matter what your diet. But when you combine clean eating with a fair amount of regular exercise, you have the perfect recipe for optimal health, happiness, and longevity.

CLEAN VS. CLEANSE

Be sure not to confuse the term "Clean" in clean eating with "Cleanse." These days, a cleanse usually refers to a short-term detox or elimination diet that is extremely calorie-restrictive and does not promote lasting weight loss or healthy habits. Detox and juice cleanses are a popular trend and can be very enticing due to their drastic promises. While cleanses have their own specific place and purpose (mainly to shed a few pounds very quickly), they should not be considered viable options for long-term wellness or sustainable weight loss.

Clean eating, on the other hand, is a mindful and healthy approach to food choices and overall wellness. It's not a short-term magic bullet, but rather an eating philosophy that focuses on increasing awareness of food and its effects on the body.

Food Groups

Clean eating is not a deprivation diet. There are certainly some foods and ingredients that are best to avoid—and we'll talk more about those coming up—but let's focus instead on all the delicious and nutritious foods you can and will be eating. It's a common misconception that healthy food is boring. I'll show you in the recipe chapters how clean eating goes way beyond salads and smoothies and is super tasty, filling, and family-friendly. To start, let's look at the different categories of foods that are the building blocks of clean eating and should make up most of your meals:

Fruits and Vegetables

Don't be shy; there isn't a bad one in the bunch! Fill your plates with plenty of fresh vegetables and fruits. In fact, aim for a plate at least half-full of non-starchy vegetables with your meals, and at least two servings of fruit per day. If you're not sure how to get your veggies in at breakfast, start by adding spinach or kale to a smoothie or scrambled eggs.

Lean Protein

Chicken, fish, eggs, and lean beef are all examples of good protein choices, but don't stop there. Leafy greens, whole grains, and dairy also provide significant amounts of protein. If you can, choose organic and grass-finished or grass-fed meats. Choosing high-quality meats that are ethically raised and sourced is a great way to feed our bodies well and take charge of what's in our food.

Whole Grains and Legumes

Loaded with fiber and protein, whole grains and legumes also play an important role in a healthy diet. Choose whole grains like quinoa, oats, or barley, and legumes such as beans, peas, lentils, and chick-peas. Whole-grain breads and pasta can be included sparingly, but pay close attention to labels. Terminology can be deceiving: Labels like "whole-wheat," "multi-grain," and "all-natural" are common but misleading, as these items often contain a whole host of additives, sugars, and preservatives. Sprouted breads and tortillas are a good substitute.

Nuts, Seeds, and Oils

Nuts and seeds are great for snacking, since they are convenient and portable, but be sure to choose raw varieties that haven't been processed with sugar or other artificial ingredients—you can always roast them yourself.

Healthy oil options include avocado oil, olive oil, and sesame oil. Stay away from vegetable oils and canola oil, which are heavily processed and very high in inflammatory omega-6 fatty acids. Let me re-emphasize that not all fats are bad. Fat actually plays a very important role in our diet and should not be avoided altogether. Your body needs fat to assist in absorbing vitamins and uses fat as energy throughout the day. Healthy fats promote heart health and help you feel satiated in between meals.

SUSTAINABILITY: HOW CLEAN EATING HELPS THE ENVIRONMENT

When you eat clean, you do your body a favor for sure, but you're likely helping the planet as well. Eating locally and seasonally is a great way to reduce your carbon footprint. Local farmers often try to grow produce with a minimum of chemicals, such as pesticides. And think about food transport. The produce you buy at a farmers' market probably arrived on a truck that came straight from the farm. Now consider the produce that came from another country. Maybe it sat on a ship, then a train, then a series of trucks. Shipping our food long distances contributes to air and water pollution, and that food loses freshness and nutritional strength along the way.

Likewise, processed food contains chemicals and requires more energy sources to produce. It is also often highly packaged, producing large quantities of non-recyclable waste on our already overburdened planet.

Finally, it is widely agreed upon that by decreasing our meat intake and eating more plant-based foods, we lessen the drain on many valuable natural resources.

YOUR WEIGHT LOSS JOURNEY

As you begin to cut out processed food and refined sugar, eat mindfully, and regularly move your body, you'll likely see weight loss as a natural byproduct. In this section, we'll explore some strategies for shifting from a "dieting" mindset to one that focuses on a commitment to lifelong healthy habits that often result in sustainable weight loss.

Food Is Your Friend

Emotional eating is a real thing. So often, food (especially the unhealthy kind) is used as a tool to soothe, reward, relieve stress, or distract from challenging times. Of course, food is delicious and should absolutely be enjoyed and celebrated when appropriate. I'll never argue that.

The problem lies in the unhealthy patterns that form when other coping mechanisms are not in place to handle stressful times. Most of us don't turn to kale and cauliflower as comfort food. Consequently, unhealthy choices over time can wreak havoc on our weight, digestion, and cardiac health.

Sometimes we eat simply out of habit. We see food, we eat it. Sound familiar? Eating mindlessly without awareness of what we're eating can occur when we're bored or looking for a distraction, or even just because others around us are eating.

The trick to breaking these patterns? Shift your thinking and redefine your relationship with food. I love the maxims "food is fuel" and "food is medicine." Being mindful when eating is a great first step to changing your relationship with food. This may include taking a moment to ponder, "Am I really hungry?" and if the answer is yes, asking yourself, "Will this food fuel my body?" Eat slowly, savoring each bite, and take time to sit and enjoy your food instead of rushing through your meal or standing over the sink to eat it—can you relate?

It's easy to see why we should eat better and cut out the junk. Food holds great power; at its worst, the negative health effects are numerous, but at its best, food can provide energy, help fight disease, and increase mood and longevity. Even so, you may be thinking, it's not that easy. To that, I say, just start! With small steps, as you begin to feel better, gain more energy, and notice other changes in your body, the day-to-day struggle to make positive choices will ease and you'll soon find yourself making healthy decisions naturally.

Understanding Calories and Portion Control

In the introduction phase of a clean eating lifestyle, it's essential to look at quantity as well as quality. If you've been eating the standard American diet—that is, extra-large portions and high in calories—shifting to smaller, healthier meals may be a challenge at first. Until your new healthy habits take hold, it will be important to keep an eye on portion sizes and overall calorie intake, at least for the next 28 days.

So, what exactly is a calorie? In simple terms, calories are energy. Nutritionally speaking, they are the units of energy coming from food that our body (brain, muscles, systems, and cells) needs to function. For weight loss to happen, we should aim for a caloric deficit (taking in fewer calories than we expend). If weight loss is your immediate goal, 1,500 calories per day for women and 2,000 calories per day for men is a good starting point. While this will vary depending on your current weight and level of activity, these guidelines are the standard for losing weight at a healthy rate (about 1 pound per week). Every individual is different and every situation unique, so the number of pounds lost will vary greatly from person to person on this 28-day plan.

That all said, calorie counting is usually associated with a "diet mind-set," which is something we're trying to avoid when adopting a clean eating lifestyle. As you slowly make positive changes by following the 10 clean eating principles (page 5), your caloric intake will be naturally regulated and weight loss or maintenance will likely follow. Here's why: Eating whole foods that are nutrient-dense and rich in fiber, protein, and healthy fats encourages satiety. This means you'll feel full longer, which will decrease the urge to snack. And as you form a new relationship with food by upping your mental game, mindless emotional eating will subsequently become a thing of the past.

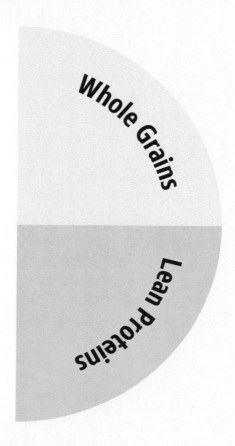

ALL CALORIES ARE NOT CREATED EQUAL

Counting calories alone doesn't work to facilitate weight loss, because ultimately it depends on where those calories come from. Take a handful of nuts versus a handful of crackers. Crackers contain simple carbs, which are quickly digested and converted to energy, often creating a surplus, which gets added to the body's fat stores and leads to weight gain. Nuts, on the other hand, contain a high amount of protein and fiber, and therefore require extra time and energy (calories) to digest, making us feel full longer and contributing to that calorie deficit we talked about.

Ultimately, quality and quantity are both important pieces of the puzzle. I find it's best to pay attention to, but be careful not to obsess over, calorie counts and instead focus on choosing nutrient-dense foods.

Identify Bad Habits

Have you been down the weight-loss path before, only to be derailed or not achieve your goals? Maybe you achieved a short-term goal, but didn't sustain the weight loss over time. Chances are that at the root of these unsuccessful attempts is a pattern of behavior or something tangible that can be corrected with the right mind-set. A little self-reflection will help you assess your negative habits honestly. Here are some common stumbling blocks I hear all the time from my readers:

There's no time. Let's face it, life gets crazy and chaotic. If you're like me, on any given day or week, you can be running in a million different directions. To avoid those last-minute desperation trips through the drive-thru, make a meal plan at the beginning of each week and invest some time on the front end prepping a few dinner ingredients, lunches, or snacks for the week ahead. A little prep goes a long way—you'll feel accomplished, prepared, and ready to tackle even the busiest of days. There's no need for desperate take-out measures when you're armed with a ready-made meal in your fridge or snack in your bag.

I frequently eat out. Not only does eating out encourage impulsive and indulgent food choices, it makes it more difficult to track exactly what you're eating. Unless you have accurate knowledge of the ingredients used by the restaurant, it's so much healthier to prepare your own meals at home. It also saves big time on your budget.

I attend lots of social gatherings. Have you ever found yourself at a social event where eating is expected but the food options are not the best? I challenge you to stop and think, take other people's expectations away from the equation, and really question if you want or need to eat what is in front of you. Step away from the buffet and focus instead on the people and the event at hand. Alternatively, eat before the event and arrive with a full stomach so you're not tempted.

Setting Goals

As you begin to focus on this new way of eating, it can help to set some intermediate goals to help keep things on track. We talked about shifting your
mind-set and tackling counterproductive habits, and this is a good place to put
that into practice.

First, identify a few areas needing improvement that will contribute to your
overall goal of adopting a clean eating lifestyle or losing weight. An example
list might look like this:

- Drinking soda
- Late-night noshing
- Struggling with a sweet tooth
- Eating as a stress reducer

Then set small goals around those behaviors and track your progress. Your
goals might include things like:

- Stop bringing soda into the home and drink water with fruit or herbs instead.
- Don't eat after 7:00 p.m. (except special occasions once a month).
- Buy berries to enjoy when the sweet tooth strikes.
- Do 10 minutes of kickboxing or yoga as a response to stress.

The habit tracker template in chapter 3 (page 41) is perfect for this.

I recommend setting multiple smaller goals that are simple to implement
and track. You'll feel accomplished as you tackle each baby step and be more
likely to want to continue. To help with this process, use the SMART strategy
of setting goals:

Specific. Be precise about what you want to achieve; for example, "increase
water intake" or "eat veggies at every meal." "Be healthier" is an example of
a non-specific goal with vague meaning.

Measurable. Attach a number to the goal. For example, "I will drink 80 ounces
of water every day."

Attainable. Your goals should be doable, not crazy pipe dreams. Again, try setting multiple small milestones that are reasonable. You'll see the results more
quickly and will be more likely to continue on your overall path to wellness.

Relevant. Will the goals you've set help you achieve your overall desired outcome? For example, if your ultimate desired outcome is to lose 15 pounds, will
your small goals contribute to that?

Timely. Your goals should have a time limit, like 28 days!

Clean Out and Stock Up

Use the following list to begin stocking your pantry and refrigerator with nutrient-dense foods.

♦ Vegetables:

Asparagus

Beets

Bell peppers

Broccoli

Brussels sprouts

Carrots

Cauliflower

Celery

Cucumbers

Eggplant

Garlic

Green beans

Kale

Lettuce (all varieties)

Mushrooms

Onion

Potatoes (all varieties)

Radishes

Spinach

Squash (all varieties)

Tomatoes (fresh
  and canned)

Zucchini

♦ Fruits:

100-percent fruit juice
  (no sugar added)

Apples

Bananas

Berries (all varieties)

Cantaloupe

Cherries

Dates

Grapefruit

Grapes

Honeydew melon

Kiwis

Mangos

Oranges

Peaches

Pears

Pineapple

Plums

Watermelon

♦ Healthy Fats:

Avocado oil

Coconut oil

Coconut milk (full-fat)

Extra-virgin olive oil

Olives

Sesame oil

◆ Nuts and Seeds (unsalted):

Almonds	Hemp seeds	Pistachios
Cashews	Macadamia nuts	Pumpkin seeds
Chia seeds	Nut butters (no	Sunflower seeds
Flaxseed	sugar added)	Walnuts
Hazelnuts	Pecans	

◆ Beans and Legumes:

Black beans	Kidney beans	Peas
Black-eyed peas	Lentils	Pinto beans
Chickpeas	Lima beans	White beans

◆ Whole Grains:

Barley	Jasmine rice	Quinoa
Brown rice	(white rice is	Whole rolled oats
Farro	minimally processed,	Whole-grain
	so use sparingly)	or sprouted bread
		(such as Ezekiel)
		Whole-grain pasta

◆ Condiments/Seasonings/Flours:

Almond flour	Cassava flour	Mustard
Arrowroot powder	Cocoa powder	Spices and herbs
Broth and/or	Coconut flour	(dried or fresh)
stock (recipes on	Ketchup	Tahini
page 163 or	(recipe on page 151	Tapioca powder
low-sodium	or store-bought	Vinegar
store-bought)	with no added sugar)	(all varieties)

◆ Meats/Protein:

Bison	Fish and shellfish	Lean beef
Chicken	(cod, tuna, whitefish,	Pork (lean cuts,
Eggs	halibut, tuna,	unprocessed)
	mahi-mahi, salmon,	Turkey
	shrimp, etc.)	Venison

♦ **Dairy:**

Cheese (without additives and not pre-shredded)	Cottage cheese (full-fat)	Greek yogurt (plain)
	Full-fat milk	Milk (full-fat)
	Ghee	Nut milks (unsweetened)

FOODS TO CUT DOWN

Store-bought condiments: Unfortunately, most of your favorite store-bought bottled condiments (ketchup, salad dressing, barbecue sauce, etc.) will not meet clean eating guidelines. Check those labels. You'll likely find loads of sugar, hydrogenated vegetable oils, and other preservatives. If the product contains high-fructose corn syrup or lists sugar as one of the first two ingredients, contains unrecognizable ingredients or more than five ingredients, or contains vegetable/canola oils, it's really got to go, because it's not doing you any favors. But check out chapter 10 (page 149) for plenty of easy, no-fuss recipes for making your own delicious, clean condiments.

Natural sweeteners: Honey, pure maple syrup, and coconut sugar are very minimally processed compared to their refined sugar counterparts but should still be used in moderation.

Dairy: Generally, most dairy is fine. Full-fat dairy products without additives are best, as lower-fat varieties are more processed. When purchasing cheese, buy blocks and shred them yourself. Stay away from all pre-shredded cheeses (even Parmesan), as they contain anti-caking agents. Avoid sweetened yogurt and instead go for plain Greek yogurt—you can add your own berries, if you like.

Processed meat products: Avoid most hot dogs, packaged deli meats, and some store-bought breakfast meats (check labels for added sugar and preservatives). If purchasing a processed meat product, look for uncured versions containing no nitrates.

FOODS TO ELIMINATE

Packaged convenience foods: Often containing excessive amounts of refined sugar, flour, and very few "real" ingredients, packaged convenience foods and snacks should be avoided. Examples include pretzels and snack mixes, granola bars, fruit snacks, crackers, most breakfast cereals, cookies, and snack cakes.

Pre-packaged meals (frozen or not) and canned soups: Pre-made meals may be labeled as "healthy," "diet," or "low-fat," but in reality, they are nothing more than poor-quality processed ingredients, usually artificially flavored and containing lots of sodium and additives.

Sugary beverages: Examples include soda, juices with added sugar, sweetened coffee and teas, and energy drinks. Don't be fooled by "energy-boosting" and "vitamin-enhanced" claims on labels. When in doubt, check the ingredient list.

Refined white sugar and artificial sweetener as an ingredient: On labels, this can appear as high-fructose corn syrup, sucrose, dextrose, cane sugar, fructose, glucose, and lactose, to name a few. Unfortunately, you'll even find it in surprising places like pasta sauce, broth, salad dressing, spice blends, even canned fruits and vegetables—another good reason to read labels and check ingredient lists.

Vegetable and canola oils: Vegetable oils are highly processed and, when consumed in excess, can contribute to inflammation in the body. Hydrogenated oils are also high in trans fats, which are associated with an increased risk of chronic disease. Examples to avoid include vegetable oil, canola oil, corn oil, soybean oil, sunflower oil, and margarine. This is actually a super easy category to comply with, since there are plenty of wonderful oils on page 15 that you can enjoy without ever feeling deprived.

Refined flour: All-purpose white and wheat flours are highly processed and bleached, stripping away all nutritional value. Like refined sugars, refined flour interferes with blood sugar regulation—you can essentially consider refined flour empty calories. It is also high in gluten, a protein found in wheat that can be difficult to digest and causes health concerns in some people. Opt for the flours listed on page 16, which are every bit as useful and delicious for cooking, baking, and thickening.

Other artificial food ingredients and chemicals: This is a broad category, but it's important to be able to identify and avoid undesirable ingredients like preservatives, harmful additives, emulsifiers, and food dyes in the foods that you purchase. Some common terms to look for on ingredient lists include artificial flavors, natural flavors (really!), artificial food color, nitrates, yeast extract, propylene glycol, olestra, and trans fats/partially hydrogenated vegetable oils. Fortunately, by eating a diet of whole ingredients including fruits, vegetables, quality protein, and healthy fats, you will naturally avoid these processed ingredients.

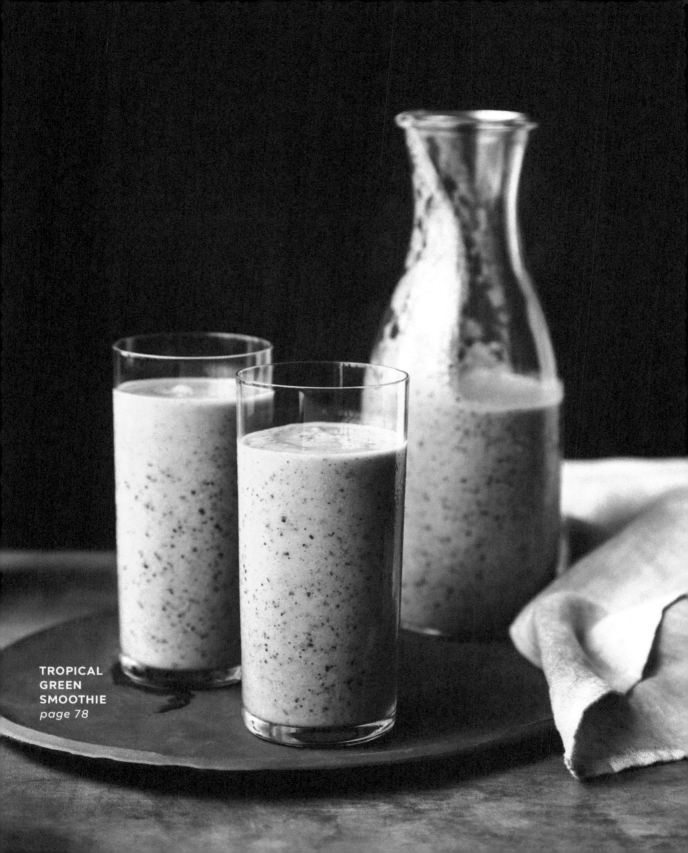

TROPICAL
GREEN
SMOOTHIE
page 78

CHAPTER TWO

EXERCISE

If there's one thing that health experts agree on, it's that physical activity is an absolutely essential component of a healthy lifestyle. A clean eating journey may begin with a shift in food and diet, but regular exercise is equally important to achieving any wellness and weight-loss goals. This section will provide tips for successfully establishing a routine that works for you.

MAKE THE MOST OF YOUR WORKOUTS

"But I hate working out. It's such a chore!" Or, "I have no time to exercise," and "Gym memberships are too expensive." I hear these excuses on a regular basis. Let me clarify that regular exercise doesn't have to mean spending hours at the gym, pouring sweat in misery. Just as clean eating focuses on making food choices that are sustainable over time, choosing an exercise routine should involve realistic options that are maintainable and even enjoyable.

To make the most of your workouts and optimize your potential for weight loss, focus on the following seven tips for success:

1. **Choose activities that you enjoy.** Don't force yourself to take up running if it's not your thing. Even if you think you despise exercising, chances are there are some activities you will prefer over others, and they may even become favorites. Explore your options, find something that resonates, and start there.

2. **Find a workout buddy.** Whether it's a daily walk with a friend or weekly workouts at home with your spouse, you will greatly increase your chances of success by having an accountability partner to help you stay on track.

3. **Add variety to your workouts.** Try a yoga class, a new walking route, or some dance moves in your kitchen! You'll be less likely to get stuck in an exercise rut if you mix it up.

4. **Take care of you.** Rest days and plenty of stretching (especially after a workout) are necessary for muscle recovery if you are new to regular exercise. Pace yourself and don't overdo it. It's okay to back off a bit and build intensity gradually.

5. **Incorporate gentle movement daily.** Our bodies are meant to move and flex, not sit all day! Take short breaks to walk or wiggle to decrease sedentary time and improve overall health.

6. **Track your progress.** A habit chart, fitness app, or wearable fitness tracker can add that extra bit of motivation.

7. **Start small.** That first step is so important! You'll quickly work your way up to longer sessions and increased intensity. We'll explore some exercises that are basic enough for a beginner but can be modified by simply increasing the weight and number of repetitions.

Set a Routine

If exercise isn't already a part of your daily routine, you may be wondering how you're going to fit it into your schedule and maintain it over time, especially alongside a new eating plan. This plan makes it realistic and easy to establish and follow a set routine with meals and exercise that will take you through the next 28 days and beyond.

Don't fall into the common trap of setting unrealistic lofty goals and expectations. By implementing a basic plan and setting intermediate goals, exercise will become a feel-good habit just like eating clean.

The following exercises can be performed at home with minimal or no equipment. If you own a set of dumbbells and a pair of walking shoes, you can easily adopt this routine. Dumbbells come in a wide variety of weights, but a good place to start might be with a 5- or 8-pound set for women or an 8- to 10-pound set for men. Try them out in the store first.

These exercises cover both cardio training and strength training. Neither category is more important than the other; rather, a balanced combination will ensure optimal results. As you settle into your new eating habits, you will likely begin to feel more energized throughout the day and ready to take on more, but to start, here are a few helpful tips:

♦ **Choose the optimal time for you.** Pick a time of day that works best with your schedule and personality. For example, if you've never been a morning person, you probably don't want to attempt 5:00 a.m. workouts.

♦ **Pencil it in.** When it comes to setting goals, I am 10 times more likely to follow through if it's written down in a list or on my calendar. Make exercise a priority like you would a doctor's appointment or work meeting. Build a 30-minute slot for exercise into your day just as you would for a favorite hobby—your future self will thank you.

♦ **Recruit a partner.** You'll achieve greater success when someone is cheering you on, and vice versa. Find and inspire like-minded people to join you on this journey. Make it a rule to regularly check in with each other to keep the momentum going. At the very least, make it known to the important people in your life that you are committed to this new lifestyle, and hopefully they will support your endeavors.

EXERCISE MYTHS

**There are plenty of unfounded theories surrounding exercise.
Holding on to them can hold you back from achieving your goals. Here are a few:**

`MYTH`

Cardio training is better than strength training.

Both are important, but strength training (light weight-lifting and resistance training) is especially crucial for building muscle mass. Greater muscle mass increases metabolism, resulting in more calories burned, even when your body is at rest.

`MYTH`

No pain, no gain.

Soreness after exercise only means a significant amount of stress was applied to the muscle tissue. A good workout can have a great impact even without next-day soreness, especially if you're using proper recovery techniques like stretching and extra hydration. But while soreness is fine, stop if any exercise causes pain—this is your body sending you a message.

`MYTH`

Lots of sit-ups will get rid of belly fat.

Sorry, but it's impossible to pick and choose specific areas of the body to trim fat through basic exercises. Sit-ups may strengthen core muscles, but they won't exclusively impact belly fat. You will, however, reduce your overall body fat by including a combination of cardio and strength training in your exercise plan.

`MYTH`

I won't see results if I don't spend hours in the gym.

Even 15 or 20 minutes per day is far better than no exercise at all. Especially when combined with diet change, adding any amount of consistent exercise to your week has major health benefits.

CARDIO AND BODY WEIGHT EXERCISES

Cardio

♦ **Walking.** Brisk walking, whether outdoors or on a treadmill, is an excellent way to get moving and raise your heart rate without putting extreme stress on the joints and muscles.

♦ **Jogging/Running.** If you want to take your walks to the next level, start with a slow jog and work up to a faster pace. Jogging and running are cardio training at its best if you're ready for the challenge.

♦ **Swimming.** Find a local pool and swim some laps. Swimming is one of the most effective exercises for the whole body and is especially easy on the joints.

♦ **Biking.** Bike riding isn't just for kids. Biking is a wonderful choice for cardio training and is a fun activity the whole family can enjoy.

♦ **Jumping jacks/High knees.** Especially when used in combination with some of the other activities on this list, a few minutes of old-school jumping jacks or high knees can really get the heart pumping.

Core

♦ **Plank.** A classic move for the core, the plank position engages the abdominal and surrounding muscles. Start by getting into a pushup position but bend your elbows and rest your weight on your forearms, forming a straight line from your shoulders to your ankles. Contract your abs and hold the position for 30 to 60 seconds at a time, or as long as you can.

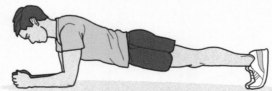

- **Hip crossover.** Lie face-up on the floor with your arms straight out from your sides, palms facing up. Raise your legs off the floor so your hips and knees are bent at a 90-degree angle as if sitting in a chair. Lower your legs to one side as far as you can go, while keeping your shoulders on the floor and your core engaged (tightened). Bring your legs back to the middle and repeat on the other side. Continue alternating the movement from side to side.

- **Reverse crunch.** The reverse crunch targets your hip flexors and obliques. Lie face-up with arms at your sides, palms down. With a slight bend in your knees, raise your hips off the floor, crunching your buttocks inward. Hold the pose, then slowly lower your legs until they almost touch the floor, keeping the same bend in your knees. Repeat as many times as desired.

Lower Body

- **Dumbbell lunges.** Stand with your feet hip-width apart, holding dumbbells at your sides. Step forward with one leg, lowering it until your front knee is bent and your rear knee is nearly touching the floor. Hold and push back up to starting position, then repeat on the other leg. Make sure you're keeping your upper body upright for proper execution.

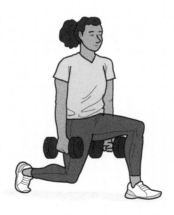

♦ **Deadlift/Row.** Hold a pair of dumbbells at arm's length in front of your hips. Bend at the hips and lower your torso into a bent-over position. Keeping your back straight and head/neck aligned with the back, pull the dumbbells up to the sides of your torso in a rowing movement, keeping your torso still. Reverse the movement to bring the dumbbells to the starting position. Repeat.

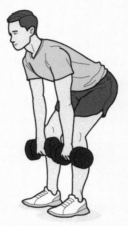

♦ **Squats.** Stand with your feet shoulder-width apart and your arms straight out in front of your body at shoulder level. Bend your knees and lower your body as far as you can go, while keeping your torso upright and arms out straight. Stick your butt out and keep your knees directly above your toes. Slowly push back up to the standing position. Repeat.

Upper Body

♦ **Hammer curl and press.** With your feet shoulder-width apart, hold a pair of dumbbells at your sides, palms facing inward. Curl the dumbbells up in front of your body toward your shoulders and press them above your head until arms are straight. Lower your arms in the reverse motion and repeat.

♦ **Push-ups.** Start on all fours with your hands slightly wider than shoulder-width apart. Keep your body in a straight line from head to ankles with your feet close together, engaging your abs and glutes. Lower your body, bending your elbows out toward the sides, until your chest nearly touches the floor, then push back up to starting position and repeat. If this move is too difficult, you can start out by doing push-ups with your knees on the floor.

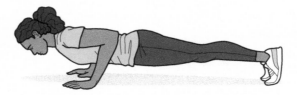

♦ **Shoulder press.** With your feet shoulder-width apart, hold the dumbbells at your sides. Bring the dumbbells to ear level with elbows bent and palms forward. Press the dumbbells up and over your head until arms are straight. Reverse the movement to return to start position and repeat.

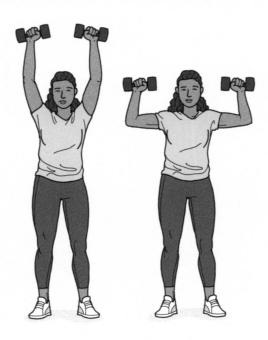

◆ **Lateral raise.** With your feet shoulder-width apart, hold the dumbbells at your sides with palms facing inward. Raise your arms up to shoulder level, keeping arms straight, forming a T with your body. Hold for 1 second and slowly lower to starting position. Repeat.

Full Body

◆ **Thrusters (push press).** Standing with your feet shoulder-width apart, bend your elbows and hold the dumbbells at your shoulders with your palms facing each other. Lower into a squat position until the tops of your legs are parallel with the floor. Push back to a standing position, simultaneously pushing the dumbbells directly over your shoulders so your arms are straight up. Lower the dumbbells back to the starting position. Repeat.

◆ **Burpees.** Start in a standing position with your feet about twice shoulder-width apart. Lower to a squat position, place your hands on the floor, and kick your feet backward, landing in a push-up position. Keep your core engaged and jump your feet back up towards your hands, landing back in a squat position, then push up to standing position. For a more advanced version, add a jump at the end of the move. Repeat.

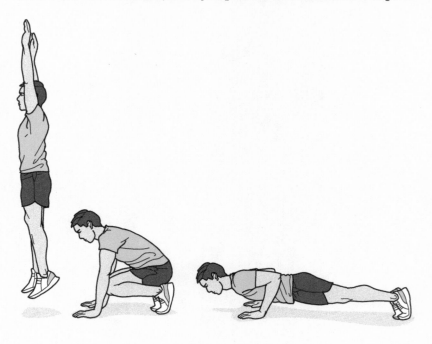

♦ **Mountain climber.** Begin in a push-up position with your arms completely straight. Lift one foot off the floor and bring the knee forward close to the chest. Return to the starting position and repeat with the other leg. Continue this move, quickly alternating your legs while keeping your body in a straight line with your abdominals engaged.

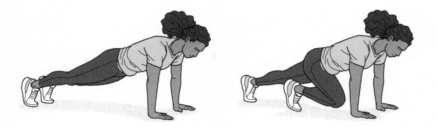

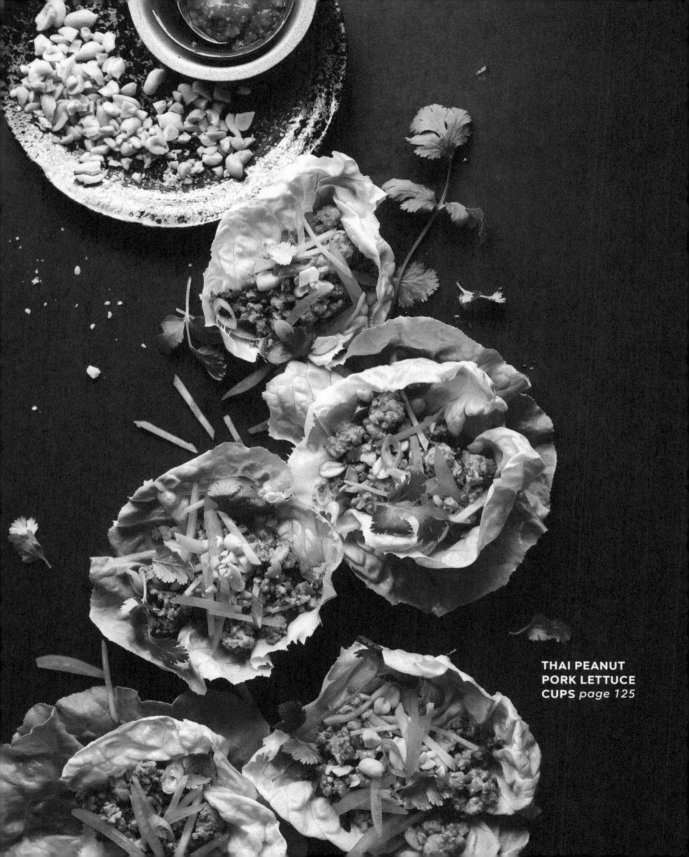

THAI PEANUT
PORK LETTUCE
CUPS *page 125*

CHAPTER THREE

THE 28-DAY PLAN

Congratulations! You've learned all about the foundations of clean eating and the numerous benefits to adopting this lifestyle. As you embark on this exciting new journey, remember that planning and preparation are key. All the tools you will need to implement a complete plan for the next 28 days are provided in this chapter, including detailed weekly menus, prep and shopping lists, exercise routines, and tips for continued success well beyond the next four weeks.

PANTRY, REFRIGERATOR, AND FREEZER STAPLES

Proper planning includes stocking your pantry and refrigerator so you'll always have ingredients and options at your fingertips. The following lists are not all-inclusive, but rather a general guide to the ingredients you will be using regularly:

♦ Pantry Staples

Almond butter

Almond flour

Arrowroot powder

Avocado oil

Baking powder

Baking soda

Beans, canned and dried (black, garbanzo, pinto, white, etc.)

Broth (low-sodium vegetable broth or chicken or beef stock, or Basic Homemade Broth/Stock, page 163)

Brown rice

Canned tomatoes (crushed, diced, and whole)

Cocoa powder

Coconut milk

Coconut oil, unrefined

Cooking spray, olive oil

Dates, pitted

Dried herbs and spices (basil, cayenne, chili powder, cinnamon, cumin, dill, freshly ground black pepper, garam masala, garlic powder, ginger, marjoram, mustard powder, nutmeg, onion powder, oregano, parsley, rosemary, sage, smoked paprika, turmeric)

Flaxseed, ground

Ghee

Honey

Hot sauce

Lentils, dried

Maple syrup (pure)

Nuts (almonds, cashews, peanuts, walnuts, etc.)

Oats, whole rolled

Olive oil, extra-virgin

Olives, canned or jarred

Peanut butter, natural

Quinoa

Salt (kosher and sea)

Sesame oil

Soy sauce, tamari, or soy sauce replacement like coconut aminos

Tahini

Tomato paste

Vanilla extract (pure)

Vinegars (apple cider, red wine, rice, and white)

♦ Refrigerator Staples

Butter, unsalted

Cheeses (not pre-shredded)

Eggs, large

Garlic, minced

Greek yogurt, plain, full-fat

Mustard (Dijon and yellow)

♦ Freezer Staples

Blueberries

Cauliflower rice

Green beans

Mango

Peas

Pineapple

Strawberries

Vegetable medleys (no sauces)

Vegetable "noodles"

Other favorite frozen fruits and vegetables

Week One

LET'S GET STARTED! This first week will be all about establishing routines, trying delicious new recipes, and incorporating whatever daily movement you've chosen.

To begin, take a few moments to review the following meal plan. You'll want to set aside some time each week for grocery shopping and prepping your meals. The few hours you spend now to plan your week will result in time saved during those busy work days—not to mention the health and money savings you'll enjoy by not having to resort to convenience foods or desperation take out. I recommend using scraps from produce to make your own stock or broth, but these shopping lists factor in the necessity of purchasing store-bought for time. If purchasing pre-made, keep an eye out for the low-sodium option.

This meal plan aligns with a 1,500 calorie per day diet, which is the standard daily caloric intake for women that will yield a weight loss of 1 pound per week. Some men may want to increase portion size by about 25 percent for the same results. Depending on your starting point, current activity level, and immediate goals, you may want to adjust your daily caloric intake slightly by increasing or decreasing portion sizes or number of snacks.

This first week, as you get used to the plan, you may find these dietary changes and routines overwhelming at times. This is perfectly normal. Don't demand too much of yourself. You are making significant strides by even opening this book. Embrace the whole process, even the ups and the downs, and remember that your new habits will gradually take hold—that's why it's a 28-day plan.

Meal Plan

	Breakfast	Lunch	Dinner	Snacks
Monday	Supreme Pizza Frittata Muffins (page 73) Piece of fruit	Curried Chicken Salad with Apples (page 89) over greens	Rosemary-Dijon Pork Tenderloin with Roasted Potatoes and Carrots (page 129)	2 to 3 snacks per day ***Suggestions:*** 2 Nutty Cranberry Oat Bites (page 132)
Tuesday	Tropical Green Smoothie (page 78) 1 egg (scrambled or hardboiled)	Leftover Rosemary-Dijon Pork Tenderloin with Roasted Potatoes and Carrots	Shrimp Tacos with Cilantro-Lime Slaw (page 112)	1 cup veggies and Greek Yogurt Dill Dip (page 160) Small piece of fruit with almond butter
Wednesday	Leftover Supreme Pizza Frittata Muffins Piece of fruit	Leftover Curried Chicken Salad with Apples over greens	Turkey Sloppy Joes (page 110) Baked sweet potato Steamed broccoli	
Thursday	Tropical Green Smoothie (page 78) 1 egg (scrambled or hardboiled)	Leftover Turkey Sloppy Joes	Cauliflower Fried Rice (page 94)	
Friday	Leftover Supreme Pizza Frittata Muffins Piece of fruit	Leftover Curried Chicken Salad with Apples over greens	Stovetop Flank Steak Fajitas (page 123) with Party Guacamole (page 158) and Fresh Salsa (page 150)	
Saturday	Cinnamon Oat Waffles (page 71) Piece of fruit	Leftover Stovetop Flank Steak Fajitas	Loaded Baked Potato and Cauliflower Soup (page 83) Crunchy Almond Broccoli Slaw (page 137)	
Sunday	Tropical Green Smoothie (page 78) 1 egg (scrambled or hardboiled)	Leftover Loaded Baked Potato and Cauliflower Soup and Crunchy Almond Broccoli Slaw	Citrus-Herb Roasted Whole Chicken with Quick Gravy (page 109) Creamy Cauliflower-Potato Mash (page 141) Steamed green beans Apple Crisp (page 143)	

Prep Ahead

- Supreme Pizza Frittata Muffins
- Curried Chicken Salad with Apples
- Salad dressing of choice
- Greek Yogurt Dill Dip
- Nutty Cranberry Oat Bites (optional snack)
- Veggie snack tray (optional snack)
- Homemade Vegetable Broth/Stock (page 163)

Shopping List

Produce

Red onion (1)	Baby carrots (1 lb.)	Cilantro (1 bunch)
Yellow onions (2)	Bell peppers (3)	Dill (1 bunch)
Baby red potatoes (1 lb.)	Broccoli (1 head)	Rosemary (1 bunch)
Russet potatoes (1 lb.)	Cauliflower (2 heads)	Apple (1 medium)
Sweet potatoes (4)	Green beans (1 lb.)	Avocados (3)
Kale (1 bunch)	Mushrooms (8 oz.)	Bananas (3)
Salad greens (10 oz.)		Lemon (1 medium)
Broccoli slaw (1 [12-ounce] bag)	Veggies for snacking (cucumber, celery, peppers, carrots, broccoli, etc.)	Lime (2 small)
Coleslaw mix (1 [14-ounce] bag)		

Meat, Poultry, Fish

Boneless, skinless chicken breast (1 pound)	Raw deveined shrimp (1 pound)	Pork tenderloin (2 pounds)
Whole chicken (3 to 4 pounds)	Ground pork or Italian sausage (1 pound)	Flank steak (1 pound)
Ground turkey (1 pound)		

continued ▶

Refrigerated/dairy

Eggs, large (2 dozen)

Parmesan cheese, not pre-shredded (4 ounces)

Plain Greek yogurt (8 ounces)

Frozen

Cauliflower rice (2 [12-ounce] bags)

Mango (6 ounces)

Pineapple (6 ounces)

Peas and carrots (8 ounces)

Pantry

Diced tomatoes (1 [14-ounce] can)

Full-fat coconut milk (1 [14-ounce] can)

Tomato sauce (1 [8-ounce] can)

Chicken or Vegetable Broth (or Homemade Broth/Stock, see page 163) (32 ounces)

Tomato paste (1 [4-ounce] can)

Slivered almonds (2 ounces)

Oats, whole rolled (1 [32-ounce] package)

Natural crunchy peanut butter (4 ounces)

Raw walnuts (1 ounce)

Dried cranberries (1.5 ounces)

Flaxseed (0.5 ounces)

Avocado or olive oil (1 [24-ounce] bottle)

Your Exercise Routine

Cardio Workouts

Four 30-minute cardio workouts each week will get your heart pumping and your blood flowing. In this first week, beginners may choose to start with shorter sessions and gradually work up to 30 minutes at a time in subsequent weeks. You can reference the list of examples on page 26 or choose any other cardio workout you enjoy (spin class, sports, etc.) that fits your current comfort level (such as walking for a beginner or running for a more advanced workout).

Strength Training

You'll want to complete a minimum of two to three strength training workouts each week to build up your strength and metabolism—awesome for losing weight and feeling great. If you are a beginner, start with two days per week and add a third day of strength training in weeks three and four or when you feel ready. Choose exercises (one for beginners and two for advanced) from each muscle group (see page 26) and complete three sets of 10 to 12 repetitions.

Rest Days

Enjoy your days off, but take time to incorporate some gentle movement throughout the day. This can include gentle stretching, yoga, or meditation—a treat for sore muscles and a wonderful stress-buster to boot. Choose stretches that target different muscle groups and always hold your stretches for a minimum of 10 to 30 seconds to get the maximum benefit.

Exercise Tracker

I've provided an exercise tracker for you to keep track of your routine. Just fill in the following plan with your choice of cardio and strength training exercises from page 26. Keep it fun by varying the exercises from week to week. As you begin to feel stronger, you're likely to be inspired to incorporate additional exercises from each muscle group—go for it!

M	T	W	TH	F	SAT	S
Cardio	**Cardio**	**REST**	**Cardio**	**REST**	**Cardio**	**REST**
	Core		**Core**			
	Lower Body		**Lower Body**			
	Upper Body		**Upper Body**			
	Full Body		**Full Body**			

Habit Tracker

There may be other healthy habits you want to prioritize and track, such as drinking at least eight glasses of water each day or getting eight hours of sleep at night. Use the following chart each week as a tool for tracking your progress in the areas that matter most to you over the next 28 days.

Habit	M	T	W	TH	F	SAT	S
Drank 8 glasses of water		X		X	X		X

Week
Two

AS YOU MOVE INTO WEEK TWO, continue building your clean foods IQ. The best way to do this is by familiarizing yourself with healthy foods, ingredient lists, and nutrition labels. You'll want to allow yourself a leisurely trip through the grocery store so you can take the time to read the labels of common packaged convenience foods like salad dressing, granola bars, and boxed cereal. Compare them to the pantry items you are purchasing. Reading food labels is an awesome habit to form, because nutrition and ingredient lists on the back dispel all the myths brought on by clever advertising tricks on the front—remember, the facts are on the back.

Be patient with yourself as you continue with this plan. Focus on what motivated you to take up clean eating in the first place, especially if doubts begin to creep in. Every day, every clean food choice, every lunge is a step toward a healthier you.

Meal Plan

	Breakfast	Lunch	Dinner	Snacks
Monday	Overnight Oats (page 70) Chicken-Apple Sausage Patties (page 75)	Mason Jar Cobb Salad (page 90) Creamy Butternut Squash Soup (page 82)	Garlic-Ginger Pork and Broccoli Stir-Fry (page 128) Cauliflower rice	2 to 3 snacks per day *Suggestions:* Veggies with 2 tablespoons Creamy Hummus (page 161) Baked Granola (page 134) ½ cup plain Greek yogurt with fruit and a drizzle of honey
Tuesday	Berry-Spinach Smoothie (page 77) 1 egg (scrambled or hardboiled)	Leftover Mason Jar Cobb Salad Leftover Creamy Butternut Squash Soup	Easy Enchilada Quinoa Skillet (page 102)	
Wednesday	Overnight Oats Leftover Chicken-Apple Sausage Patties	Leftover Easy Enchilada Quinoa Skillet	Blackened Salmon with Cool Tomato-Cucumber Relish (page 114) Tomato and Avocado Salad (page 86)	
Thursday	Berry-Spinach Smoothie 1 egg (scrambled or hardboiled)	Mason Jar Cobb Salad (page 90) Leftover Creamy Butternut Squash Soup	Olive-Feta Sliders with Tzatziki Sauce (page 122) Balsamic Roasted Vegetables (page 139)	
Friday	Overnight Oats Leftover Chicken-Apple Sausage Patties	Leftover Mason Jar Cobb Salad Leftover Creamy Butternut Squash Soup	Slow Cooker Chicken Tikka Masala (page 107) Cauliflower rice	
Saturday	2 eggs 1 serving of fruit	Leftover Slow Cooker Chicken Tikka Masala	Asparagus and Mushroom Frittata (page 97) Mixed greens w/olive oil and balsamic vinegar	
Sunday	Berry-Spinach Smoothie 1 egg (scrambled or hardboiled)	Leftover Asparagus and Mushroom Frittata Mixed greens	Skillet Shepherd's Pie (page 121) Quick Berry Sorbet (page 146)	

Prep Ahead

- Overnight Oats
- Chicken-Apple Sausage Patties
- Mason Jar Cobb Salads
- Creamy Butternut Squash Soup
- Veggie snack tray (optional snack)
- Creamy Hummus (optional snack, page 161)
- Baked Granola (optional snack, page 134)
- Homemade Vegetable Broth/Stock (page 163)
- Salad dressing of choice

Shopping List

Produce

Yellow onions (2)

Red onion (1)

Russet potatoes (1 pound)

Asparagus (1 pound)

Bell peppers (2)

Broccoli (1 large head)

Brussels sprouts (8 ounces)

Butternut squash (1 large, about 16 ounces)

Carrots (1 pound)

Cauliflower (2 heads)

Cherry tomatoes (16 ounces)

English cucumber (1)

Mushrooms (8 ounces)

Romaine lettuce (10 ounces)

Scallions (1 bunch)

Spinach (10 ounces)

Zucchini (1 medium)

Veggies for snacking

Cilantro (1 bunch)

Apple (2 medium)

Avocado (1)

Lemon (1 medium)

Lime (1 small)

Meat, Poultry, Fish

Boneless, skinless chicken breast (2 lbs.)

Ground chicken (1 lb.)

Salmon fillets (16 ounces)

Pork loin chops (1 lb.)

Uncured bacon (1 lb.)

Ground beef or sirloin (2 lbs.)

Refrigerated/dairy

Eggs, large (2 dozen)

Feta cheese (1 ounce)

Plain Greek yogurt
(8 ounces)

Frozen

Cauliflower rice
(2 [10-ounce] bags)

Blueberries (10 ounces)

Strawberries (10 ounces)

Pantry

Beef and Chicken broth
(or Homemade Broth/
Stock, page 163)
(24 ounces)

Full-fat coconut milk
(2 [13.5-ounce] cans)

Black beans
(1 [15-ounce] can)

Chickpeas
(1 [15.5-ounce] can)

Quinoa (1 [16-ounce] bag)

Fire-roasted diced toma-
toes (1 [14.5-ounce] can)

Kalamata olives (1 ounce)

Coconut flakes (3 ounces)

Raw almonds (1 ounce)

Tahini paste (1 [16-ounce]
container)

Your Exercise Routine

Cardio Workouts

Get that blood pumping—complete a minimum of four 30-minute cardio workouts this week! If you are a beginner, you may choose to start with shorter sessions and gradually work up to 30 minutes in duration. Your cardio workout doesn't have to be vigorous, but it should be intense enough to elevate your heart rate. Just a little cardio will generate feel-good hormones as you simultaneously strengthen your heart and lungs.

Strength Training

Vary your strength training workouts from day to day and week to week—this will help you diversify the muscles you strengthen. Try pairing some of last week's preferred exercises with a few new ones. Choose one or two exercises from each muscle group and complete three sets of 10 to 12 repetitions. Your muscles should begin to tire toward the end of each set. If not, you can probably stand to increase your weight or repetitions. Aim for a minimum of two to three strength training workouts this week. Strength training increases bone density, important for long-term health. And remember—muscle equals metabolism, so you'll burn more calories.

Rest Days

If regular exercise is new to you, it may be helpful to incorporate yoga on your rest days. Yoga is wonderful for centering yourself and increasing flexibility and can be a useful tool for preventing injury. To get started, grab a book from the library or access one of the many free Internet resources (see page 167) and learn a few poses.

Exercise Tracker

Keep track of your routine by filling in the following plan with your favorite cardio and strength training exercises from page 26. Keep things fresh by varying the exercises from week to week. As you begin to feel stronger, add on exercises from each muscle group.

M	T	W	TH	F	SAT	S
Cardio	**Cardio**	REST	**Cardio**	REST	**Cardio**	REST
	Core		**Core**			
	Lower Body		**Lower Body**			
	Upper Body		**Upper Body**			
	Full Body		**Full Body**			

Habit Tracker

Forming new habits takes time. While you're waiting to see the rewards of your efforts, remember that your small daily actions are making a big difference in the long run. With every day that you prioritize a healthy habit, you're taking another step toward achieving your goals.

Habit	M	T	W	TH	F	SAT	S
Drank 8 glasses of water		X		X	X		X

Week
Three

BY NOW, YOU'RE PROBABLY FINDING a groove with your new routine. Keep doing what you're doing—forge on, stay positive, and appreciate that you are making choices for a healthier you. Amp up your workouts if you're feeling ready.

Meal Plan

	Breakfast	Lunch	Dinner	Snacks
Monday	Buffalo Chicken Hash Brown Egg Bake (page 76) Piece of fruit	Chickpea Salad Power Bowls with Olives and Feta (page 87)	Cashew Chicken Skillet (page 106) Cauliflower rice	2 to 3 snacks per day *Suggestions:* ½ cup Quick Refrigerator Pickles (page 135) and olives Veggies Stovetop popped popcorn with sea salt (1 cup)
Tuesday	Banana-Blueberry Oatmeal Muffin (page 72) 1 egg (scrambled or hardboiled)	Leftover Cashew Chicken Skillet Piece of fruit	Mini Marinara Meatloaves (page 120) Baked Broccoli Fritters (page 138)	
Wednesday	Leftover Buffalo Chicken Hash Brown Egg Bake Piece of fruit	Leftover Chickpea Salad Power Bowls with Olives and Feta	Sausage, White Bean, and Kale Stew (page 85)	
Thursday	Leftover Banana-Blueberry Oatmeal Muffin 1 egg (scrambled or hardboiled)	Leftover Sausage, White Bean, and Kale Stew Piece of fruit	Garlic-Herb Salmon with Potato and Asparagus en Papillote (page 116)	
Friday	Leftover Buffalo Chicken Hash Brown Egg Bake Piece of fruit	Leftover Chickpea Salad Power Bowls with Olives and Feta	Sheet-Pan Shrimp and Chicken Jambalaya (page 111) Cauliflower rice	
Saturday	2 eggs Fruit	Leftover Sheet-Pan Shrimp and Chicken Jambalaya	Veggie-Loaded Lentil Chili (page 103) Arugula salad dressed with lemon juice and olive oil	
Sunday	Soothing Mint Chocolate Smoothie (page 79) 1 egg (scrambled or hardboiled)	Leftover Veggie-Loaded Lentil Chili	Sunday Pot Roast and Root Vegetables (page 124) No-Bake Chocolate–Almond Butter Bars (page 145)	

Prep Ahead

- Buffalo Chicken Hash Brown Egg Bake
- Banana-Blueberry Oatmeal Muffins
- Chickpea Salad Power Bowls with Olives and Feta
- Salad dressing of choice
- Quick Refrigerator Pickles (optional snack, page 135)
- Veggie snack tray (optional snack)
- Homemade Vegetable Broth/Stock (page 163)

Shopping List

Produce		
Yellow onions (2 large or 4 small)	Carrots (1 pound)	Baby arugula (16 ounces)
Baby red potatoes (1 pound)	Cauliflower (1 head)	Kale (1 bunch)
Yukon gold potatoes (1 pound)	Celery (1 bunch)	Spinach (8 ounces)
Asparagus (1 pound)	Cherry tomatoes (8 ounces)	Cilantro (1 bunch)
Bell peppers (3)	English cucumber (1)	Mint (1 bunch)
Broccoli (1 head)	Parsnips (1 pound)	Rosemary (1 bunch)
	Veggies for snacking	Bananas (4)
		Lemon (1 medium)

Meat, Poultry, Fish		
Boneless, skinless chicken breast (3 pounds)	Salmon fillets (16 ounces)	Ground beef or sirloin (1.5 pounds)
Raw deveined shrimp (1 pound)	Ground pork or Italian sausage (1 pound)	Beef chuck roast (2 pounds)

Refrigerated/dairy		
Eggs, large (2 dozen)	Feta cheese (2 ounces)	Parmesan cheese, not pre-shredded (1 ounce)

continued ▶

Frozen

Cauliflower rice
(2 [10-ounce] bags)

Blueberries (4 ounces)

Stir-fry vegetable medley
(14.5 ounces)

Pantry

Kalamata olives (2 ounces)

Water chestnuts
(1 [8-ounce] can)

Chicken broth (or Home-
made Broth/Stock, see
page 163) (32 ounces)

Coconut milk, full fat
(1 [14-ounce] can)

Crushed tomatoes
(1 [28-ounce] can)

Tomato paste

Diced tomatoes
(1 [14.5-ounce] can)

Lentils (7 ounces)

White beans
(2 [15-ounce] cans)

Black beans
(1 [15-ounce] can)

Chickpeas
(1 [15-ounce] can)

Raw cashews (3 ounces)

Buffalo sauce (4 ounces)

Your Exercise Routine

Cardio Workouts

If you haven't already, this week is a good time to push yourself on the length and intensity of your cardio workouts. Shoot for four sessions of cardio, each lasting at least 30 minutes. Try a new activity this week with an open mind and attitude. Toss a football or play some basketball, head over to a skating rink, or go hiking at a nearby park. Have you ever tried geocaching? You may just surprise yourself and find a new passion.

Strength Training

Do a quick self-assessment of your strength training sessions thus far. Are you challenging yourself enough? If you didn't feel challenged in weeks one and two, add a third day of strength training and/or increase your number of repetitions per exercise. Add some new strengthening exercises this week, paying close attention to the different muscle groups you are targeting.

Rest Days

Want a real treat? Give meditation a try on your rest days. The practice of meditation is known to reduce stress and anxiety, help fight addictions, and increase mental clarity. While there are many forms of meditation, a simple five- to ten-minute session of sitting in a quiet space without distractions and focusing on your breath can be a great place to start.

Exercise Tracker

What's it going to be this week? To keep track of your routine, fill in the following plan with your choice of cardio and strength training exercises from page 26. Remember to vary the exercises from week to week. As you begin to feel stronger, dig deeper and add on some new exercises from each muscle group.

M	T	W	TH	F	SAT	S
Cardio	**Cardio**	REST	**Cardio**	REST	**Cardio**	REST
	Core		**Core**			
	Lower Body		**Lower Body**			
	Upper Body		**Upper Body**			
	Full Body		**Full Body**			

Habit Tracker

Habit trackers are effective because it can be incredibly satisfying to record your successes right in the moment. They can be a great motivator to continue, but don't beat yourself up if you miss a day. Perfection is not the goal here—instead, try to make it a personal rule to not miss two days whenever possible.

Habit	M	T	W	TH	F	SAT	S
Drank 8 glasses of water		X		X	X		X

Week Four

YOU'VE MADE IT TO THE HOME STRETCH and your routines are beginning to take root as good habits. Celebrate your progress! Along with your clean eating and exercise routines, your shopping trips and prep sessions are probably becoming second nature, too. Do you feel the difference you've made in your body? Congratulate yourself on your commitment and all that you've learned and accomplished.

Meal Plan

	Breakfast	Lunch	Dinner	Snacks
Monday	Bacon Egg Cups (page 74) Fruit	Buffalo Chicken and Ranch Lettuce Wraps (page 91)	Chicken Parmesan Meatballs (page 108) Balsamic Roasted Vegetables (page 139)	2 to 3 snacks per day *Suggestions:* Roasted Rosemary Mixed Nuts (¼ cup) 1 cup veggies with Greek Yogurt Dill Dip (page 160)
Tuesday	Tropical Green Smoothie (page 78) 1 egg (scrambled or hardboiled)	Leftover Chicken Parmesan Meatballs Roasted Balsamic Veggies	Thai Peanut Pork Lettuce Cups (page 125)	
Wednesday	Leftover Bacon Egg Cups Fruit	Leftover Buffalo Chicken and Ranch Lettuce Wraps	Slow Cooker Mini Meatball and Vegetable Soup (page 84) Green salad w/dressing	
Thursday	Tropical Green Smoothie (page 78) 1 egg (scrambled or hardboiled)	Leftover Slow Cooker Mini Meatball and Vegetable Soup	Crispy Mahi Tenders (page 113) Tomato and Avocado Salad (page 86)	
Friday	Leftover Bacon Egg Cups Fruit	Leftover Buffalo Chicken and Ranch Lettuce Wraps	Slow Cooker Chickpea and Vegetable Curry (page 98) Cauliflower rice	
Saturday	Cinnamon Oat Waffles (page 71) Chicken-Apple Sausage Patties (page 75)	Leftover Chickpea and Vegetable Curry	Avocado Tuna Salad (page 88) Tuscan Tomato–White Bean Bisque (page 99)	
Sunday	Tropical Green Smoothie (page 78) 1 egg (scrambled or hardboiled)	Leftover Avocado Tuna Salad Leftover Tuscan Tomato–White Bean Bisque	Slow Cooker Barbecue Pulled Pork Cajun-Spiced Sweet Potato Fries (page 140) Crunchy Almond Broccoli Slaw (page 137) Mango Soft Serve (page 144)	

Prep Ahead

- Bacon Egg Cups
- Buffalo Chicken and Ranch Lettuce Wraps
- Roasted Rosemary Mixed Nuts (optional snack)
- Veggie snack tray (optional snack)
- Greek Yogurt Dill Dip (optional snack)
- Salad dressing of choice
- Homemade Vegetable Broth/Stock (page 163)

Shopping List

Produce

Red onion (1)

Yellow onions (2 small)

Sweet potatoes (16 ounces)

Yukon gold potatoes (2 pounds)

Bell pepper (1)

Broccoli slaw (1 [10-ounce] bag)

Brussels sprouts (8 ounces)

Carrots (1 pound)

Cauliflower (2 heads)

Celery (1 bunch)

Cherry tomatoes (8 ounces)

Mushrooms (8 ounces)

Scallions (1 bunch)

Zucchini (1 medium)

Veggies for snacking

Boston leaf lettuce (2 heads)

Kale (8 ounces)

Salad greens (16 ounces)

Dill (1 bunch)

Cilantro (1 bunch)

Avocado (1)

Bananas (3)

Lime (2 small)

Meat, Poultry, Fish

Boneless, skinless chicken breasts (1 pound)

Ground chicken (1 pound)

Mahi-mahi fillets (1 pound)

Uncured bacon (1 pound)

Pork shoulder (3 pounds)

Ground pork (1 pound)

Ground beef (1 pound)

Refrigerated/dairy

Eggs, large (2 dozen)

Feta cheese

Parmesan cheese, not pre-shredded (2 ounces)

Plain Greek yogurt (8 ounces)

Frozen

Cauliflower rice
(1 [10-ounce] bag)

Mango (6 ounces)

Pineapple (6 ounces)

Pantry

Raw almonds (5 ounces)

Raw cashews (5 ounces)

Raw peanuts (1 ounce)

Raw pecans (5 ounces)

Crushed tomatoes
(1 [28-ounce] can)

Diced tomatoes
(2 [14-ounce] cans)

Tomato paste (1 ounce)

Whole tomatoes
(1 [28-ounce] can)

Beef broth (or Homemade
Broth/Stock, see page
163) (24 ounces)

Vegetable broth (or
Homemade Broth/Stock,
see page 163)

Chickpeas
(1 [15-ounce] can)

White beans
(1 [15-ounce] can)

Wild-caught albacore tuna
(2 [6-ounce] cans)

Water chestnuts (1 can)

Full-fat coconut milk
(1 [14-ounce] can)

Your Exercise Routine

Cardio Workouts

Keep that momentum going, and don't back down on the quality and duration of your cardio workouts this week. If you're comfortable, bump up the intensity—for example, bring a brisk walk up to a slow jog or a slow jog to a run—or just increase each session by five or 10 minutes. Try the steeper hiking trail this time—bring your camera up to the peak! These boosts will maximize the effectiveness of your workouts and speed your results, in addition to making you feel great.

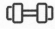

Strength Training

As with your cardio workouts, strength training should be getting easier in this fourth week, so go ahead and push yourself beyond your comfort zone. Perform at least two exercises from each muscle group, add a few new exercises you have yet to try, and increase your reps to 12 to 15 per set. Crank your best playlist and let it move you!

Rest Days

Continue to explore the joy of "me time" through yoga and meditation on your rest days, and at the very least, incorporate a short stretching session. Rest days are crucial to muscle recovery, but also important for maintaining mental clarity and remaining focused on your new goals.

Exercise Tracker

Keep keeping track! Fill in the following plan with your choice of cardio and strength training exercises from page 26. You've likely come up with great new ways to get that blood pumping.

M	T	W	TH	F	SAT	S
Cardio	Cardio	REST	Cardio	REST	Cardio	REST
	Core		Core			
	Lower Body		Lower Body			
	Upper Body		Upper Body			
	Full Body		Full Body			

Habit Tracker

Hopefully, the process of tracking certain behaviors has been a helpful visual reminder to you. You'll want to keep the momentum going, so by all means, continue tracking your goals beyond the 28 days.

Habit	M	T	W	TH	F	SAT	S
Drank 8 glasses of water		X		X	X		X

BEYOND 28 DAYS

Congratulations on the progress you've made in the last 28 days! Be proud of all your accomplishments and realize that you have taken a huge step toward reaching optimal health and wellness. Hopefully you've experienced how a clean eating lifestyle can be satisfying, energizing, and sustainable. With the tools you have acquired in the last four weeks of practical experience, you are well on your way to a robust and healthy future—for you and anyone you may be cooking for.

Now is a great time to recall your reasons for starting this journey. Do a quick goal check. Whether you aimed to cut out processed foods, lose weight, or reduce your risk of disease, understand that you have only just begun to see results. The real dividends will be realized in the months and years to come.

Maintaining Priorities

You've probably noticed a consistent message throughout this book—clean eating is a lifestyle choice, not a diet plan. While the last 28 days have been carefully designed to set you up for success, it's merely the springboard for you to use all you've learned and remain dedicated to maintaining your new habits in the long-term.

Undoubtedly, there will be good days and bad days, successes and struggles, and hopefully an increased sense of ease in your new routines. Don't beat yourself up if you falter; simply revisit your priorities, refocus, and renew your faith in yourself. You may find that certain aspects of your new lifestyle are easier to maintain than others. Follow the instincts this plan has helped you to develop and hold yourself to your own goals. Finding balance, while being mindful and intentional with your choices, will help you achieve long-term success. Unlike restrictive fad diets, you can rejoice in the fact that clean eating includes the best of both worlds—plenty of healthy food that is also totally delicious.

It may help to circle back and review the principles of clean eating (page 4) if you notice yourself slipping back into negative habits. These foundations are a good starting point when old patterns resurface. Continue educating yourself on healthy practices and the benefits of clean eating to help stay motivated. Refer to this book regularly and check out page 167 for resources to expand your knowledge of this subject.

Workouts that Don't Feel Like Workouts

Now that you've made regular exercise part of your daily routine, you may occasionally feel like ditching the dumbbells for other forms of exercise. By all means! Consider all the different ways to incorporate movement in your day by looking for new and exciting options to supplement your workouts. You'll have more fun and probably target some rarely used muscle groups in the process. Here are a few suggestions for creatively incorporating cardio and strength training into your day:

♦ **Take a family hike or bike ride.** Grab your partner, spouse, kids, or a friend and hit the trails. Meeting health goals while still enjoying quality time with family and friends is a win-win.

♦ **Pick up a sport.** From a low-impact game of tennis to advanced rock climbing, group and individual sports are an engaging and challenging way to stay active. Your local YMCA is a great resource for exploring new sports activities and fitness classes.

♦ **Do some household chores.** These tasks may not be anyone's idea of fun, but they get us moving and burn calories nonetheless. A solid house-cleaning session including vacuuming, mopping, washing windows, or scrubbing the bathroom can result in some serious calorie burn.

♦ **Get outside with yard work.** Take double advantage of being outdoors—work in your yard or clean up your block. Check off those items on your to-do list while getting active and working multiple muscle groups. Gardening, weeding, mowing the lawn, and raking leaves are all excellent choices that count as physical activity.

♦ **Dance your heart out.** Take advantage of a joyful, stress-relieving aerobic activity—dance! Join a local dance class, find a place with live music, or throw a dance party right in your own kitchen.

PRACTICES FOR ACHIEVING LONG-TERM SUCCESS

Quality Sleep and Hydration

It's no secret that a good night's sleep does wonders for our health, mood, and energy level. Do your best to get seven to eight hours of rest on a regular basis for optimal health. If falling asleep is a struggle for you, establish a nighttime routine that includes wind-down time—take a hot bath, drink a cup of herbal tea, shut off your phone, read a book, or write in a gratitude journal. Build a ritual to help quiet your brain before you attempt sleep.

Adequate hydration is a commonly overlooked cornerstone of good health. Don't neglect to provide your body with its number-one needed nutrient, water. I've found it helpful to drink a large glass of water right upon waking and then refill a large Mason jar throughout day. Proper hydration includes sipping all day, not just at meals or workouts. Your body will thank you.

Stress Management and Gentle Movement

While it's impossible to totally avoid all of life's stressors, how we handle them is well within our control. Stress plays a huge role in the development of many health issues, and the best thing you can do to keep healthy stress levels is to establish coping mechanisms for managing stress when it creeps up. Discover wholesome practices that make sense for you, such as practicing meditation, spending quality time with family and friends, getting a massage, or making time for your favorite hobby. Your mental well-being is equal to your physical health, and each impacts the other.

The concept of gentle movement simply means being conscious of our amount of daily sedentary time and incorporating movement at regular intervals. It can be difficult to recognize how much of our day is filled with activities that leave our bodies idle, like sitting at a desk, watching TV, or riding in a car or train. Some of the most preventable diseases and health issues stem from excessive sedentary time. Break up long periods of sitting time with short periods of walking, stretching, or gentle movement. A fitness tracker can be helpful for providing reminders to get up and move.

Mindfulness and Journaling

Be intentional with your food choices, from what you eat to how you eat it. Awareness of what goes into our food is the foundation of eating clean, so do your research, check nutrition labels, ask questions of your local farmers, and choose the best quality ingredients you can find. When you sit down to eat that food, take the time to focus in on each bite.

Mindfulness also means being self-aware. You know yourself best, but introspective techniques such as regular journaling can be a useful tool for noticing internal and external factors affecting your choices. Tracking your food, sleep, and exercise habits is a great way to see (and celebrate!) your progress, but it's also helpful for identifying troublesome patterns and roadblocks so you can address them. Think of a written journal or fitness app/tracker as your built-in accountability partner.

PART TWO

The Recipes

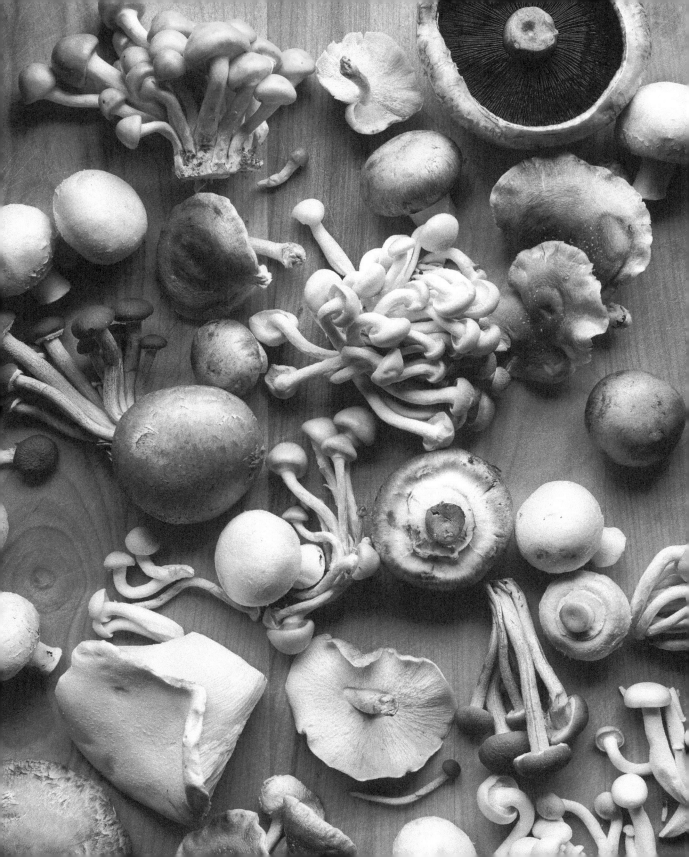

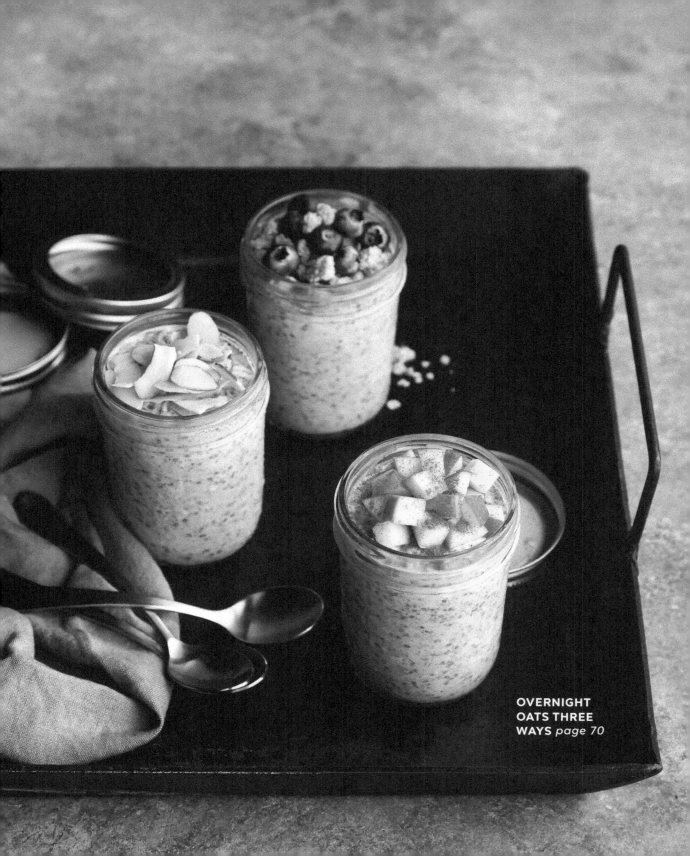

OVERNIGHT
OATS THREE
WAYS *page 70*

CHAPTER FOUR

BREAKFAST AND SMOOTHIES

Overnight Oats Three Ways

Yield: 4 servings, Prep time: 10 minutes, plus 8 hours to chill

QUICK PREP, VEGETARIAN

When busy schedules get the best of you, these Overnight Oats are great to have on hand for a quick breakfast on the go. They last a few days, so make up to four jars at a time, then customize with your choice of toppings or eat them as-is.

For the overnight oats base

2 cups whole rolled oats

2 cups unsweetened almond milk or water

1 cup plain Greek yogurt

4 tablespoons pure maple syrup

4 teaspoons chia seeds

1 teaspoon vanilla extract

1 teaspoon cinnamon

For the toppings

APPLE PIE:

¼ cup diced apples

¼ teaspoon cinnamon

COCONUT-ALMOND:
2 tablespoons flaked coconut

2 tablespoons sliced raw almonds

BLUEBERRY GRANOLA:

¼ cup fresh blueberries

2 tablespoons Baked Granola (page 134)

1. In each of 4 small Mason jars, pour ½ cup of oats, ½ cup of almond milk, ¼ cup of yogurt, 1 tablespoon of maple syrup, 1 teaspoon of chia seeds, ¼ teaspoon of vanilla, and ¼ teaspoon of cinnamon. Stir to combine.

2. Cover the jars and refrigerate overnight. Before eating, stir again, and add additional milk if the mixture is too thick. Add your choice of toppings. Store in the refrigerator for up to 5 days.

SUBSTITUTION TIP: If dairy yogurt isn't an option for you, swap it out here with your preferred type—unsweetened will work best.

PER SERVING (WITHOUT TOPPINGS): Total calories: 291; Total fat: 9g; Saturated fat: 3g; Carbohydrates: 45g; Sodium: 35mg; Fiber: 6g; Protein: 9g

Cinnamon Oat Waffles

Yield: 4 servings, Prep time: 10 minutes, Cook time: 10 minutes
30 MINUTES OR LESS, DAIRY-FREE, QUICK PREP, VEGETARIAN

Oats are a wonderful, delicious, nutrient-dense whole grain. Loaded with fiber and protein, they are also high in vitamins and minerals and are the only readily available source of avenanthramides, a powerful group of antioxidants thought to protect against heart disease. Pair these tasty waffles with Chicken-Apple Sausage Patties (page 75) and a side of fruit for a wholesome breakfast.

2 cups whole rolled oats

1 tablespoon baking powder

2 teaspoons cinnamon

½ teaspoon sea salt

2 large eggs

¼ cup melted coconut oil

1¼ cups unsweetened almond milk

½ teaspoon pure vanilla extract

Olive oil cooking spray

Pure maple syrup (optional)

Fresh berries (optional)

1. Pour the oats into a blender and pulse until finely ground.

2. Add the baking powder, cinnamon, salt, eggs, coconut oil, almond milk, and vanilla and blend until completely combined and smooth, scraping down the sides as needed.

3. Preheat a waffle iron and spray with cooking spray.

4. Pour about ⅓ cup of batter into the waffle iron (amount will depend on the size of your waffle maker).

5. Cook for 3 to 4 minutes, or until steam no longer escapes from the sides of the waffle iron.

6. Serve with pure maple syrup or fresh berries, if using.

SUBSTITUTION TIP: Any milk can be substituted for the almond milk.

PER SERVING: Total calories: 321; Total fat: 20g; Saturated fat: 13g; Carbohydrates: 30g; Sodium: 756mg; Fiber: 5g; Protein: 9g

Banana-Blueberry Oatmeal Muffins

Yield: 12 muffins, Prep time: 10 minutes, Cook time: 18 minutes
30 MINUTES OR LESS, DAIRY-FREE, NUT-FREE, QUICK PREP

Muffins are an ideal grab-and-go breakfast or snack. This recipe demonstrates how easy it can be to swap out white sugar and white flour with healthier alternatives. Ripe bananas lend plenty of sweetness to these muffins, while oat flour replaces refined flour, adding a boost of fiber and protein.

Olive oil cooking spray

3 ripe bananas

⅓ cup melted coconut oil

1 large egg, beaten

1½ cups oat flour (see Ingredient tip)

1 teaspoon baking soda

1 teaspoon baking powder

1 teaspoon cinnamon

1 cup fresh or frozen blueberries

1. Preheat the oven to 350°F. Spray a 12-cup muffin tin with cooking spray.

2. In a large bowl, mash the bananas. Stir in the coconut oil and egg.

3. In a separate bowl, combine the oat flour, baking soda, baking powder, and cinnamon, stirring well.

4. Add the dry ingredients into the banana mixture, stirring to combine. Gently fold in the blueberries.

5. Fill the muffin cups about half-full with batter. Bake for 18 minutes.

6. Let the muffins cool for about 10 minutes before removing from the tin.

INGREDIENT TIP: You can usually find oat flour in the baking aisle of your grocery store, but you can easily make your own. Simply pulse whole oats in a blender until finely ground into a flour-like consistency.

PER SERVING: Total calories: 147; Total fat: 8g; Saturated fat: 5g; Carbohydrates: 19g; Sodium: 153mg; Fiber: 3g; Protein: 3g

Supreme Pizza Frittata Muffins

Yield: 12 muffins, Prep time: 10 minutes, Cook time: 20 minutes

30 MINUTES OR LESS, NUT-FREE

Mini frittata muffins make an excellent choice for breakfast on the go. This version offers a fun way to enjoy your favorite pizza toppings for breakfast. They're endlessly versatile, so feel free to find new flavor combinations or use up leftover meats and clean out that veggie drawer.

Olive oil cooking spray

1 cup cooked crumbled Italian sausage (for homemade, see Ingredient tip, page 85)

⅓ cup finely diced green bell pepper

⅓ cup chopped mushrooms

¼ cup finely diced onion

12 large eggs, beaten

⅓ cup grated Parmesan cheese

Dried oregano

1. Preheat the oven to 375°F. Coat the cups of a 12-cup muffin tin with cooking spray.

2. Layer equal amounts of the sausage, bell pepper, mushrooms, and onion in the bottoms of the muffin cups.

3. Pour the eggs into each cup, filling about two-thirds full.

4. Sprinkle the Parmesan cheese and dried oregano on the top of each muffin cup.

5. Bake for 15 to 20 minutes, until the eggs are set. Remove from the oven and allow to cool for 10 minutes. To release, run a knife around the inside of each muffin cup before removing the muffins from the tin. Enjoy warm.

COOKING TIP: You can make these muffins ahead, then freeze them in an airtight, freezer-safe container. Reheat when ready to eat by placing in the microwave for 1 to 2 minutes or by warming in a toaster oven or skillet.

PER SERVING: Total calories: 121; Total fat: 8.6g; Saturated fat: 3.1g; Carbohydrates: 1.3g; Sodium: 219mg; Fiber: 0.1g; Protein: 9.7g

Bacon Egg Cups

Yield: 6 servings, Prep time: 5 minutes, Cook time: 20 minutes

**5 INGREDIENTS OR LESS, 30 MINUTES
OR LESS, DAIRY-FREE, NUT-FREE, QUICK PREP**

Here's a quick and easy two-ingredient, make-ahead breakfast. This recipe can be easily doubled to fit a bigger family's needs. Serve these protein-loaded egg cups with one of the smoothies in this chapter for a well-rounded meal.

Olive oil cooking spray

½ pound uncured bacon (6 strips)

6 large eggs

Sea salt

Freshly ground black pepper

1. Preheat the oven to 400°F. Spray a 6-cup muffin tin with cooking spray.

2. Place a strip of bacon in each muffin cup, around the outside edges. Bake for 10 minutes.

3. Remove from the oven and crack an egg into each bacon cup. Season with salt and pepper and bake for an additional 10 to 12 minutes, until the eggs are set.

4. Once cooled, remove the bacon egg cups from the pan. Store in an airtight container in the refrigerator for up to 3 days, reheating as desired.

INGREDIENT TIP: Bacon as a "clean" food is somewhat controversial. Cured bacon (with added nitrites) should be avoided, but you can still enjoy bacon in moderation if you look for an uncured, sugar-free version.

PER SERVING: Total calories: 102; Total fat: 7.3g; Saturated fat: 2.6g; Carbohydrates: 0.4g; Sodium: 216mg; Fiber: 0g; Protein: 8.3g

Chicken-Apple Sausage Patties

Yield: 10 patties, Prep time: 10 minutes, Cook time: 15 minutes

**5 INGREDIENTS OR LESS, 30 MINUTES OR LESS,
ALLERGEN-FRIENDLY, DAIRY-FREE, NUT-FREE, QUICK PREP**

Store-bought breakfast sausage often contains additives and extra sodium, but you can easily make your own with just a few ingredients. These scrumptious patties are the perfect mix of sweet and savory and are freezer-friendly, too.

1 pound ground chicken

½ cup finely diced apples (peeled or unpeeled)

1 teaspoon Poultry Seasoning Blend (page 164)

1 teaspoon sea salt

Pinch cinnamon

2 tablespoons extra-virgin olive oil, divided

1. Line a plate with paper towels. Set aside.

2. In a bowl, combine the ground chicken, apple, poultry seasoning, sea salt, and cinnamon. Mix well and form into patties.

3. In a large sauté pan or skillet over medium-high heat, heat 1 tablespoon of olive oil. Working in batches, add the patties to the skillet, cooking 3 to 4 minutes per side, until browned and cooked through. Add more oil to the pan as needed to prevent sticking.

4. Transfer the cooked patties to the paper towel–lined plate to drain. Serve warm.

COOKING TIP: To freeze, let the patties cool completely, then place on a baking sheet lined with wax paper. Flash-freeze the patties by placing the baking sheet in the freezer for about 20 minutes. Transfer the patties to a large freezer-safe container. Remove when ready to eat, and warm in the microwave or in a stovetop skillet.

PER SERVING: Total calories: 108; Total fat: 7.6g; Saturated fat: 1.6g; Carbohydrates: 1.4g; Sodium: 268mg; Fiber: 0.2g; Protein: 8.4g

Buffalo Chicken Hash Brown Egg Bake

Yield: 12 servings, Prep time: 10 minutes, Cook time: 40 minutes

DAIRY-FREE, NUT-FREE

This savory casserole with classic buffalo chicken flavors can be made ahead and reheats beautifully for a quick breakfast. Enjoy this dish for lunch or dinner as well, topped with a drizzle of Creamy Ranch Dressing (page 155) and sliced scallions.

Olive oil cooking spray

1 tablespoon extra-virgin olive oil

½ cup finely diced carrots

½ cup finely diced celery

½ cup finely diced onion

½ cup Avocado Oil Mayonnaise (page 153)

⅓ cup hot sauce

2 cups shredded potatoes

2 cups shredded cooked chicken (see Ingredient tip, page 89)

1 teaspoon sea salt

6 large eggs, beaten

1. Preheat the oven to 350°F. Prepare a 9-by-13-inch baking dish with cooking spray.

2. In a sauté pan or skillet over medium-high heat, warm the olive oil. Add the carrots, celery, and onion and cook for 5 minutes, or until softened.

3. In a large bowl, whisk the mayonnaise and hot sauce until well combined.

4. Add the vegetable mixture, shredded potatoes, chicken, and salt to the bowl and stir to combine.

5. Fold in the beaten eggs and spread the mixture in the prepared baking dish. Bake for 40 minutes.

INGREDIENT TIP: Homemade mayonnaise is a cinch to make, but if you prefer to purchase your mayonnaise from the store, look for versions made with olive oil or avocado oil that do not contain sugars and additives.

PER SERVING: Total calories: 181; Total fat: 13.4g; Saturated fat: 2g; Carbohydrates: 3.6g; Sodium: 570mg; Fiber: 1g; Protein: 11.6g

Berry-Spinach Smoothie

Yield: 1 serving, Prep time: 5 minutes

**5 INGREDIENTS OR LESS, 30 MINUTES OR LESS, ALLERGEN-FRIENDLY,
DAIRY-FREE, NUT-FREE, QUICK PREP, VEGAN/VEGETARIAN**

This smoothie is a nutrition powerhouse packed with fiber, antioxidants, protein, and healthy fats. Berries and spinach are known for their anti-inflammatory properties, so enjoy this wonderful recovery tool to supplement your new workout routine.

¾ cup frozen blueberries

4 large fresh or frozen strawberries

½ large, ripe banana

1 cup packed spinach leaves

1 tablespoon ground flaxseed

¾ cup water (or more, as needed)

1. Combine the blueberries, strawberries, banana, spinach, flaxseed, and water in a blender and blend until completely smooth and creamy.

2. Serve immediately.

INGREDIENT TIP: Don't let your fresh spinach go to waste—make frozen spinach cubes! Any time you have extra, put the spinach leaves and water in a blender and purée. Pour the mixture into ice cube trays and freeze. Adding frozen spinach cubes to smoothies for a serving of veggies will be a breeze.

PER SERVING: Total calories: 184; Total fat: 4.4g; Saturated fat: 0.4g; Carbohydrates: 38g; Sodium: 26.5mg; Fiber: 8.7g; Protein: 4g

Tropical Green Smoothie

Yield: 1 serving, Prep time: 5 minutes

5 INGREDIENTS OR LESS, 30 MINUTES OR LESS, ALLERGEN-FRIENDLY, DAIRY-FREE, NUT-FREE, QUICK PREP, VEGAN/VEGETARIAN

Did you know that kale is one of the most nutrient-dense foods on the planet? Just one cup of raw kale contains vitamins, A, C, and K, folate, omega-3 fatty acids, and nearly 3 grams each of protein and fiber. If cooked kale isn't your thing, you can reap its benefits by tossing some into this delicious tropical fruit smoothie.

½ **large ripe banana**

½ **cup frozen pineapple**

½ **cup frozen mango**

1 cup packed kale leaves

¼ **avocado**

1 cup water

1. Combine the banana, pineapple, mango, kale, avocado, and water in a blender and blend until completely smooth and creamy.

2. Serve immediately.

SUBSTITUTION TIP: Swap the water for coconut water to provide an extra dose of electrolytes and a boost of tropical flavor.

PER SERVING: Total calories: 254; Total fat: 7.7g; Saturated fat: 1.1g; Carbohydrates: 46.6g; Sodium: 34.2mg; Fiber: 9.3g; Protein: 4.5g

Soothing Mint Chocolate Smoothie

Yield: 1 serving, Prep time: 5 minutes

5 INGREDIENTS OR LESS, 30 MINUTES OR LESS, DAIRY-FREE, QUICK PREP, VEGAN/VEGETARIAN

Sweet and refreshing, this smoothie can be paired with a protein source like hardboiled eggs for a quick breakfast or enjoyed on its own as a quick, sweet treat.

1 large very ripe banana

1 cup crushed ice

1 tablespoon cocoa powder

3 tablespoons unsweetened almond milk

1 cup spinach leaves

4 or 5 fresh mint leaves

1. Combine the banana, ice, cocoa powder, almond milk, spinach, and mint in a blender and blend until completely smooth and creamy.

2. Serve immediately.

SUBSTITUTION TIP: Try substituting coconut milk for the almond milk.

PER SERVING: Total calories: 148; Total fat: 1.8g; Saturated fat: 0.6g; Carbohydrates: 35.8g; Sodium: 59.5 mg Fiber: 6.5g; Protein: 3.7g

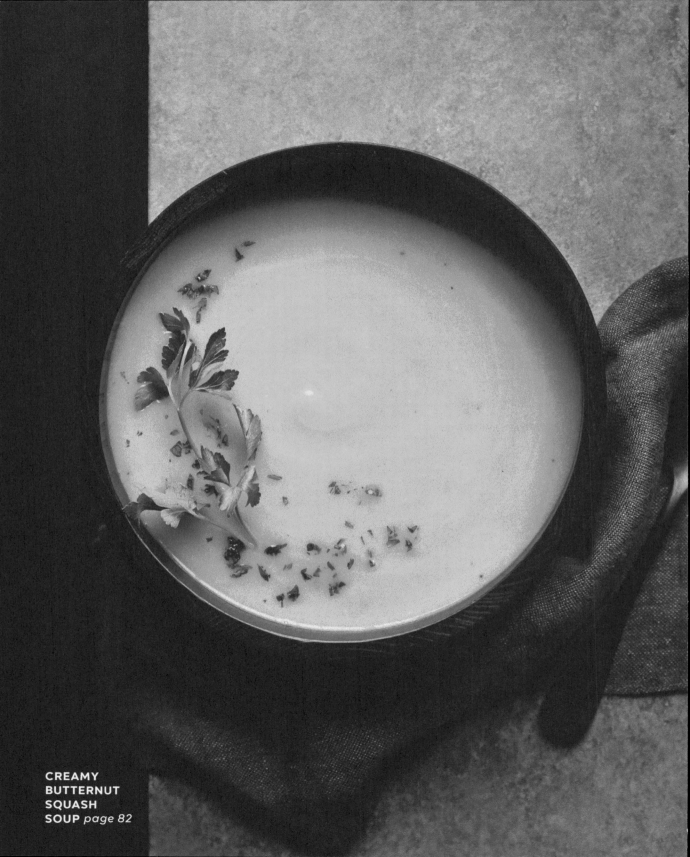

CREAMY
BUTTERNUT
SQUASH
SOUP *page 82*

CHAPTER FIVE

SOUPS, SALADS, AND SANDWICHES

Creamy Butternut Squash Soup

Yield: 8 cups, Prep time: 10 minutes, Cook time: 25 minutes
ALLERGEN-FRIENDLY, DAIRY-FREE, QUICK PREP, VEGAN/VEGETARIAN

Butternut squash is loaded with vitamin A and is super delicious! This homey and nutritious soup is perfect with a salad on the side. It also reheats beautifully, so make it ahead for lunch all week.

1 tablespoon extra-virgin olive oil

¾ cup diced carrots

1 small yellow onion, diced

4 cups cubed fresh or frozen butternut squash

2 cloves garlic, minced

4 cups Basic Homemade Broth (page 163)

⅓ cup full-fat coconut milk

Sea salt

Freshly ground black pepper

1. In a large pot over medium-high heat, warm the oil. Add the carrots and onion and sauté for 3 to 4 minutes or until soft.

2. Add the squash and garlic and continue to cook uncovered, stirring frequently, for another 3 to 4 minutes.

3. Pour in the broth and bring to a boil. Reduce the heat and simmer for 15 minutes.

4. Remove from the heat. Purée the soup with an immersion blender or carefully purée in batches in a standard blender (cover with a towel to prevent spattering).

5. Stir in the coconut milk and add salt and pepper to taste.

COOKING TIP: Invest in an immersion blender to make creamy soups a breeze. They are relatively inexpensive and perfect for working with wet ingredients.

PER SERVING: Total calories: 88; Total fat: 3.6g; Saturated fat: 1.8g; Carbohydrates: 14.4g; Sodium: 248mg; Fiber: 3.5g; Protein: 1.3g

Loaded Baked Potato and Cauliflower Soup

Yield: 7 cups, Prep time: 10 minutes, Cook time: 25 minutes

ALLERGEN-FRIENDLY, DAIRY-FREE (WITHOUT CHEESE), ONE-POT, QUICK PREP

Cauliflower hides out in this rich and creamy soup that tastes just like a baked potato. Despite its decadent taste, this soup is healthy for you—plus, it's gluten-free and even dairy-free if you leave out the cheese. Toppings optional.

1 tablespoon extra-virgin olive oil

1 medium head cauliflower, roughly chopped

1 small yellow onion, chopped

2 stalks celery, chopped

3 small Yukon gold potatoes, chopped

2 teaspoons minced garlic

4 cups Basic Homemade Broth (page 163)

1 cup full-fat coconut milk

1½ teaspoons sea salt

½ teaspoon freshly ground black pepper

1 strip crumbled cooked bacon (optional)

⅓ cup shredded cheddar cheese (optional)

1 scallion, chopped (optional)

1. In a large pot over medium-high heat, warm the oil. Add the cauliflower, onion, celery, and potatoes and cook for 3 to 4 minutes, stirring frequently.

2. Add the minced garlic and broth and bring to a boil. Reduce the heat and simmer uncovered for 20 minutes.

3. Using an immersion blender, purée the vegetables and broth until completely smooth. Stir in the coconut milk, salt, and pepper.

4. Serve topped with crumbled bacon, cheese, and scallions (if using).

COOKING TIP: If you like a chunkier texture to your soup, don't purée it completely in step 3. Blend the soup slightly to create a thick base but leave some of the potatoes and cauliflower chunks whole or chopped to your desired consistency.

PER SERVING (WITHOUT TOPPINGS): Total calories: 154; Total fat: 8.3g; Saturated fat: 5.5g; Carbohydrates: 19.4g; Sodium: 807.8mg; Fiber: 3.8g; Protein: 4g

Slow Cooker Mini Meatball and Vegetable Soup

Yield: 8 servings, Prep time: 10 minutes, Cook time: 4 hours

DAIRY-FREE, ONE-POT

This wholesome soup is perfect to return home to on a chilly day. Customize to your taste by using your preferred vegetables, potatoes, or ground meat.

For the soup

3 cups Basic Homemade Beef Stock (see Variation tip, page 163)

1 (14.5-ounce) can diced tomatoes

1 cup diced zucchini

1 cup diced carrots

1 cup diced Yukon gold potatoes

½ cup diced onion

2 tablespoons tomato paste

1 tablespoon Italian Seasoning Blend (page 164), or store-bought Italian seasoning

1 teaspoon minced garlic

1 teaspoon kosher salt

For the meatballs

1 pound lean ground beef

½ cup almond flour

1 large egg

1 teaspoon sea salt

1. In a slow cooker, pour in the stock, tomatoes, zucchini, carrots, potatoes, onion, tomato paste, seasoning blend, garlic, and salt and stir to combine.

2. In a large bowl, mix together the beef, flour, egg, and salt until just combined. Do not overmix. Roll into ½-inch meatballs and drop into the soup.

3. Cook on high for 4 to 5 hours or on low for 7 to 8 hours.

COOKING TIP: Save time by forming the meatballs and prepping the veggies ahead. Meatballs can be stored in an airtight container in the refrigerator for up to 24 hours or in the freezer for 3 to 4 months. If freezing, thaw in the refrigerator for 12 to 24 hours before making the soup.

PER SERVING: Total calories: 176; Total fat: 8.2g; Saturated fat: 2g; Carbohydrates: 11.7g; Sodium: 950.8mg; Fiber: 3g; Protein: 14.7g

Sausage, White Bean, and Kale Stew

Yield: 8 cups, Prep time: 10 minutes, Cook time: 20 minutes

30 MINUTES OR LESS, ALLERGEN-FRIENDLY, DAIRY-FREE, NUT-FREE, QUICK PREP

This hearty stew delivers Tuscan flair and loads of flavor. Enjoy for dinner with a side salad and portion out the leftovers for easy, make-ahead lunches.

1 tablespoon extra-virgin olive oil

1 pound turkey Italian sausage

1 cup diced carrots

1 small yellow onion, diced

2 teaspoons minced garlic

½ teaspoon red pepper flakes

4 cups Basic Homemade Broth (page 163)

2 (15.5-ounce) cans white beans (cannellini or great northern), drained and rinsed

1 cup full-fat coconut milk

2 cups kale, stems removed

1. In a large stock pot over medium-high heat, warm the oil. Squeeze the sausage from its casings into the pot and break up with a wooden spoon. Cook, stirring often, until browned, about 5 minutes. Drain and set aside.

2. In the same pot, add the carrots and onion. Cook for 3 to 4 minutes, stirring occasionally, until the vegetables begin to soften. Add the garlic and red pepper flakes, and cook, stirring frequently, for 1 minute.

3. Add the broth and beans and bring to a boil. Cover, reduce the heat, and cook for 10 minutes.

4. Stir in the sausage and coconut milk until completely combined.

5. Remove from the heat, stir in the kale, and cover for 5 minutes, until the kale is wilted.

INGREDIENT TIP: Make your own Italian sausage by browning 1 pound of ground turkey (or pork) with 1 teaspoon of Italian Seasoning blend (page 164), 1 teaspoon of sea salt, and ½ teaspoon of ground sage.

PER SERVING: Total calories: 269; Total fat: 12.2g; Saturated fat: 6.1g; Carbohydrates: 23.8g; Sodium: 593.9mg; Fiber: 5.8g; Protein: 15.9g

Tomato and Avocado Salad

Yield: 4 servings, Prep time: 10 minutes

30 MINUTES OR LESS, NUT-FREE, VEGETARIAN

Tomatoes and avocado come together for a super tasty dish, and their nutritional properties complement each other perfectly. Tomatoes contain high levels of lycopene, which is an antioxidant known as a carotenoid, believed to reduce the risk of cardiovascular disease and cancer. The healthy fat in avocados is responsible for absorption of those carotenoids in the body, making this a beautiful marriage of two delicious ingredients.

1 large ripe avocado, peeled and pitted

12 ounces multi-colored cherry or grape tomatoes

¼ cup very thinly sliced red onion

1 ounce queso blanco or feta cheese, crumbled

1 tablespoon chopped fresh cilantro

1 to 2 tablespoons freshly squeezed lime juice (juice of ½ lime)

¼ teaspoon kosher salt

1. Cut the avocado and tomatoes into equal bite-size pieces and put in a large bowl.

2. Add the onion, cheese, cilantro, lime juice, and salt and gently toss to combine. Serve promptly.

INGREDIENT TIP: I prefer cherry tomatoes for this recipe because they are bite-size and easy to chop, but other varieties of tomatoes also work well here. Just seed the tomato and squeeze out any extra juice to prevent a soggy salad.

PER SERVING: Total calories: 123; Total fat: 9g; Saturated fat: 2.1g; Carbohydrates: 9.2g; Sodium: 237mg; Fiber: 4.6g; Protein: 2.8g

Chickpea Salad Power Bowls with Olives and Feta

Yield: 4 servings, Prep time: 15 minutes

30 MINUTES OR LESS, NUT-FREE, VEGETARIAN

No need to spend $10 or more on a salad or grain bowl from a restaurant when you can make your own at home—and control the ingredients. Bold Greek flavors take this salad to another level. Briny olives, sweet tomatoes, and tangy feta deliver a beautiful balance to spicy arugula and creamy chickpeas. The vinaigrette in this recipe can be prepared and used as an all-purpose dressing for any salad.

For the dressing

⅓ **cup extra-virgin olive oil**

2½ **tablespoons freshly squeezed lemon juice**

1 teaspoon Dijon mustard

1 teaspoon honey

Sea salt

Freshly ground black pepper

For the salad

4 cups baby arugula

1 (15.5-ounce) can chickpeas, drained and rinsed

1 cup cherry tomatoes, halved

1 cup diced English cucumber

1 cup Kalamata olives, sliced

½ **cup feta cheese**

To make the dressing

Whisk the olive oil, lemon juice, Dijon mustard, honey, salt, and pepper until well combined. Alternatively, pour in a small Mason jar, seal, and shake vigorously until combined. Set aside.

To make the salad

1. Divide the arugula, chickpeas, tomatoes, cucumber, olives, and feta equally among 4 bowls or containers.

2. Serve each bowl with 1 to 2 tablespoons of dressing.

VARIATION TIP: Boost the power in these bowls even more with a scoop of quinoa, nuts, or seeds.

PER SERVING: Total calories: 386; Total fat: 27.7g; Saturated fat: 5.9g; Carbohydrates: 26g; Sodium: 472mg; Fiber: 6.2g; Protein: 10g

Avocado Tuna Salad

Yield: 4 servings, Prep time: 10 minutes

5 INGREDIENTS OR LESS, 30 MINUTES OR LESS, DAIRY-FREE, NUT-FREE, QUICK PREP

Bursting with flavor, this colorful salad is packed with protein and healthy fats, a combo that will keep you feeling satisfied until your next meal. Serve over fresh greens and with a side of fruit for a deliciously balanced meal.

2 (6-ounce) cans albacore wild-caught tuna, drained

1 avocado, peeled, pitted, and diced

¼ cup thinly sliced red onion

Juice and zest of 1 lemon

1 tablespoon extra-virgin olive oil

1 teaspoon sea salt

½ teaspoon freshly ground black pepper

1. Scoop the tuna into a medium bowl. Use a fork to break it into chunks.

2. Add the diced avocado, red onion, lemon juice and zest, olive oil, salt, and pepper. Toss gently.

3. Serve immediately over greens, or store in a covered container in the refrigerator for 1 to 2 days.

INGREDIENT TIP: The avocado can be diced into chunks as directed or mashed prior to mixing for a texture more like tuna salad.

PER SERVING: Total calories: 158; Total fat: 7.2g; Saturated fat: 0.9g; Carbohydrates: 5.4g; Sodium: 785mg; Fiber: 3g; Protein: 17g

Curried Chicken Salad with Apples

Yield: 2½ cups, Prep time: 20 minutes

30 MINUTES OR LESS, DAIRY-FREE

This chicken salad is the perfect recipe for weekly meal prep. Juicy chicken, warm curry spice, and sweet apples blend for a satisfying combination you can serve over greens or in a lettuce cup.

4 tablespoons Avocado Oil Mayonnaise (page 153)

1 tablespoon curry powder

½ teaspoon sea salt

2 cups shredded cooked chicken

¼ cup finely diced apples

¼ cup slivered almonds

1 tablespoon chopped fresh cilantro

Mixed greens or lettuce cups

1. In a small bowl, stir together the mayonnaise, curry powder, and salt.

2. In a large bowl, combine the shredded chicken, apples, almonds, and cilantro. Add the curry-mayo mixture and stir well to combine.

3. Serve over mixed greens or scooped into lettuce cups.

INGREDIENT TIP: To make shredded chicken, boil 2 boneless, skinless chicken breasts (about 1¼ pounds) in water for about 15 minutes, or until the chicken reaches an internal temperature of 165°F. Remove from the water and drain. Using two forks, shred the chicken to your desired consistency.

PER ½ CUP: Total calories: 256; Total fat: 17g; Saturated fat: 2g; Carbohydrates: 2.8g; Sodium: 614mg; Fiber: 1.3g; Protein: 21g

Mason Jar Cobb Salad

Yield: 4 servings, Prep time: 15 minutes

30 MINUTES OR LESS, DAIRY-FREE, NUT-FREE, QUICK PREP

One of my favorite ways to prepare for a busy week is to build lunch salads to go in Mason jars. They are convenient and perfectly layered with a rainbow of ingredients. Vary the type of greens, vegetables, dressing, and protein to make your own special version. Other delicious add-ins include cooked whole grains (quinoa, lentils, etc.), chopped nuts or seeds, and fruit.

8 tablespoons Creamy Ranch Dressing (page 155), or dressing of choice

1 cup cherry tomatoes, quartered

1 cup diced cucumber

4 hardboiled eggs, chopped

2 cups shredded cooked chicken breast (see Ingredient tip, page 89)

6 strips cooked uncured bacon, chopped

4 cups chopped romaine lettuce

1. Layer the ingredients into pint-size (or larger) Mason jars in the following order: dressing, tomatoes, cucumber, eggs, chicken, bacon, and lettuce.

2. To serve, pour a salad into a large bowl and toss to combine. If using larger Mason jars with extra room, simply shake the jar to toss the salad and eat directly from the jar.

COOKING TIP: When layering these salads, the order of ingredients matters. To prevent a soggy salad, the dressing always goes on the bottom and the lettuce on top. You can also keep the ingredients like the bacon and dressing separate until ready to serve.

PER SERVING: Total calories: 482; Total fat: 33.6g; Saturated fat: 6.2g; Carbohydrates: 4g; Sodium: 748.9mg; Fiber: 1.6g; Protein: 34.3g

Buffalo Chicken and Ranch Lettuce Wraps

Yield: 4 servings, Prep time: 10 minutes

DAIRY-FREE, NUT-FREE, QUICK PREP

Clean eating doesn't mean giving up your comfort foods. These crunchy lettuce wraps have all the flavor of buffalo chicken wings without the greasy, deep-fried element.

2 cups shredded cooked chicken (see Ingredient tip, page 89)

¼ cup Avocado Oil Mayonnaise (page 153)

1½ tablespoons hot sauce

8 to 12 Boston Bibb lettuce leaves

1 large carrot, peeled and cut into thin matchsticks

1 large celery stalk, cut into thin matchsticks

Creamy Ranch Dressing (page 155), for drizzling

1. Put the shredded cooked chicken in a bowl.

2. Add the mayonnaise and hot sauce and stir to combine well.

3. Scoop the chicken mixture into lettuce cups. Sprinkle with the carrot and celery matchsticks and a drizzle of dressing. Alternatively, divide equal portions of lettuce cups, chicken, carrots, celery, and ranch dressing among 4 containers for make-ahead lunches.

VARIATION TIP: Give this dish a new spin—skip the hot sauce, swap out the dressing for Sesame-Ginger Dressing (page 154), and sprinkle with toasted sesame seeds.

PER SERVING: Total calories: 287; Total fat: 17.3g; Saturated fat: 1.7g; Carbohydrates: 3.1g; Sodium: 610.3mg; Fiber: 1.2g; Protein: 25.2g

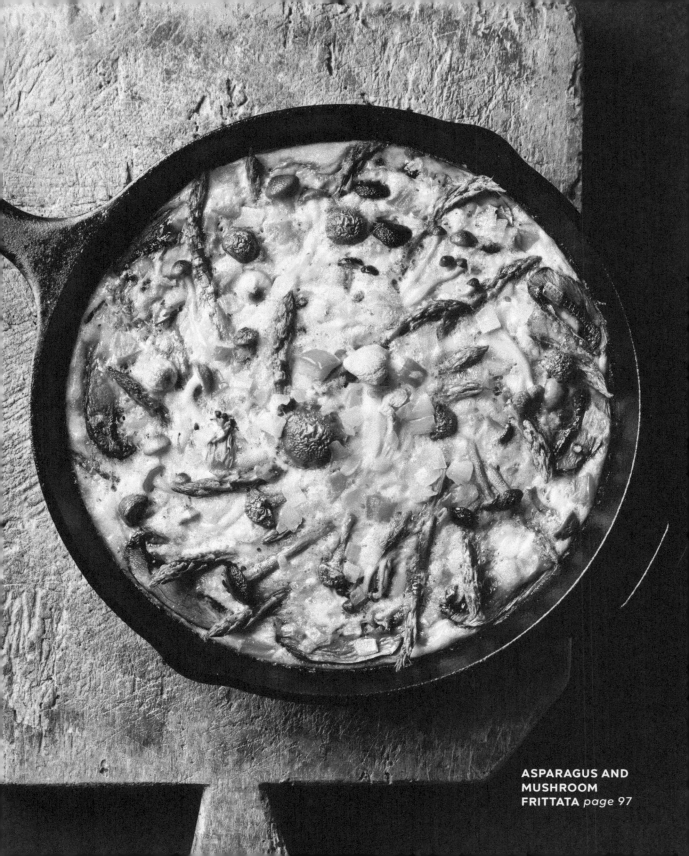

ASPARAGUS AND
MUSHROOM
FRITTATA *page 97*

MEATLESS MAINS

Cauliflower Fried Rice

Yield: 6 servings, Prep time: 5 minutes, Cook time: 10 minutes

**30 MINUTES OR LESS, DAIRY-FREE, NUT-FREE, QUICK PREP,
VEGAN/VEGETARIAN**

Look to cauliflower rice as a healthy option in all your rice dishes. Very mild in flavor, it often goes unnoticed as a substitute for white rice. Make your own or find it prepared in the freezer section. This fun recipe contains a good dose of veggies and protein and is super family-friendly.

2 tablespoons extra-virgin olive oil, plus more as needed, divided

1½ cups frozen peas and carrots

3 scallions, finely chopped

2 (12-ounce) bags frozen cauliflower rice

1½ teaspoons minced garlic

1 teaspoon grated fresh ginger

3 large eggs, beaten

½ teaspoon freshly ground black pepper

¼ cup light soy sauce

1. In a large sauté pan or skillet over medium-high heat, warm the oil.

2. Add the peas and carrots and scallions to the pan. Cook, stirring occasionally, for 3 to 4 minutes, until the vegetables begin to soften.

3. Add the cauliflower rice, garlic, and ginger, stirring well to combine. Cook for 1 minute.

4. Push the mixture to the outside edges of the pan and pour the eggs into the middle. Scramble the eggs, cooking and stirring until set, about 3 minutes.

5. Add the pepper and soy sauce, stirring all ingredients well to combine. Cook for an additional 2 to 3 minutes, adding a drizzle of oil as needed to prevent the mixture from sticking to the pan.

SUBSTITUTION TIP: If you're sensitive to soy, coconut aminos is a wonderful substitute for soy sauce. It can be found in most grocery stores and specialty health food stores.

PER SERVING: Total calories: 135; Total fat: 7.1g; Saturated fat: 1.4g; Carbohydrates: 12.4g; Sodium: 511.3mg; Fiber: 4.1g; Protein: 7.9g

Vegetable Lo Mein with Carrot Noodles

Yield: 4 servings, Prep time: 15 minutes, Cook time: 10 minutes

30 MINUTES OR LESS, DAIRY-FREE, NUT-FREE, VEGAN/VEGETARIAN

The classic take-out dish gets a makeover in this recipe. Vegetable "noodles" serve as a fun and refreshing alternative to pasta, and the homemade stir-fry sauce brings classic flavors to this dish.

12 ounces frozen carrot "noodles"

½ tablespoon extra-virgin olive oil

1 teaspoon sesame oil

2 scallions, sliced

1 red bell pepper, cut into strips

1 cup shredded Napa cabbage

1 teaspoon minced garlic

1 cup snap peas

½ cup Stir-Fry Sauce (page 157)

1. Cook the carrot noodles according to the package directions. Set aside.

2. In a large sauté pan or skillet over medium-high heat, warm the olive oil and sesame oil. Add the scallions and bell pepper to the skillet and stir-fry for 3 to 4 minutes, until the vegetables begin to soften.

3. Add the cabbage, garlic, and snap peas. Continue to cook, stirring, for an additional 2 minutes.

4. Shake or whisk the stir-fry sauce, then add the carrot noodles and sauce to the pan. Stir well and cook until the sauce thickens, about 2 minutes.

5. Serve warm.

INGREDIENT TIP: Use frozen zucchini or butternut squash noodles in place of the carrot noodles. If you own a spiralizer, you can add the vegetable noodles of your choice at step 4.

PER SERVING: Total calories: 119; Total fat: 3.8g; Saturated fat: 0.5g; Carbohydrates: 19.9g; Sodium: 649mg; Fiber: 3.5g; Protein: 2.3g

Zucchini-Mushroom Marinara Roll-Ups

Yield: 4 servings, Prep time: 15 minutes, Cook time: 25 minutes
NUT-FREE, VEGETARIAN

High in vitamins, minerals, and disease-fighting antioxidants, leafy greens are delicious as well as nutritious—especially when wrapped up in a neat zucchini package.

3 large zucchini

1 tablespoon extra-virgin olive oil, divided

4 ounces mushrooms, finely diced

3 ounces Swiss chard, chopped

1 cup ricotta cheese

1 teaspoon garlic powder

½ teaspoon sea salt

¼ teaspoon freshly ground black pepper

2 cups Marinara Sauce (page 152)

1. Preheat the oven to 400°F. Line a large baking sheet with parchment paper.

2. Trim the ends off the zucchini and cut into long, ½-inch-thick vertical slices.

3. Place the zucchini in a single layer on the prepared baking sheet. Spread ½ tablespoon of olive oil on the zucchini and roast until just tender, 10 to 15 minutes.

4. In a large sauté pan or skillet over medium-high heat, warm the remaining ½ tablespoon of olive oil. Add the mushrooms and cook for 5 to 6 minutes, stirring occasionally, until soft.

5. Add the chard and continue to cook, stirring occasionally, until wilted, about 2 to 3 minutes. Remove the mushrooms and chard from the heat.

6. In a medium bowl, combine the ricotta, garlic powder, salt, pepper, and cooked mushrooms and chard.

7. Spread 1 cup of marinara sauce in the bottom of a 9-by-13-inch baking dish.

8. Spread each zucchini slice with the ricotta mixture and carefully roll up. Place seam-side down in the baking dish.

9. Top each roll-up with a spoonful of marinara sauce. Cover with foil and bake for 15 minutes.

INGREDIENT TIP: Go for the full-fat ricotta. Low-fat counterparts of most cheeses are more processed and have fewer nutrients.

PER SERVING: Total calories: 216; Total fat: 12.7g; Saturated fat: 5.8g; Carbohydrates: 17g; Sodium: 682.6mg; Fiber: 4.6g; Protein: 14.9g

Asparagus and Mushroom Frittata

Yield: 4 servings, Prep time: 10 minutes, Cook time: 35 minutes
DAIRY-FREE, NUT-FREE, VEGETARIAN

Oven-baked frittatas can be enjoyed for any meal of the day and customized based on your favorite flavor combinations or ingredients you have on hand. While the frittata is baking, whip up a quick side salad to serve alongside this filling dish.

1 tablespoon extra-virgin olive oil, plus more for greasing the pie dish

8 ounces mushrooms, sliced

½ cup diced yellow onion

8 ounces asparagus, woody stems removed and cut into 1-inch pieces

½ cup chopped tomatoes

1 teaspoon sea salt

½ teaspoon freshly ground black pepper

8 large eggs, beaten

1. Preheat the oven to 350°F. Grease a 9-inch pie dish and set aside.

2. In a large sauté pan or skillet over medium-high heat, warm the oil. Add the mushrooms and onion and cook, stirring occasionally, for 3 to 4 minutes, until they begin to soften.

3. Add the asparagus and continue to cook, stirring occasionally, for 2 to 3 minutes. Stir in the tomatoes and season with salt and pepper. Spread the vegetables evenly in the pie dish.

4. Pour the eggs over the vegetable mixture. Bake for 20 to 25 minutes, until the eggs are set. Remove from the oven and serve warm.

VARIATION TIP: Add ¼ cup of feta cheese to the mix for an extra flavor boost or substitute chopped spinach, diced bell peppers, sliced zucchini, or chopped broccoli for the vegetables.

PER SERVING: Total calories: 213; Total fat: 13.5g; Saturated fat: 3.8g; Carbohydrates: 8.2g; Sodium: 729.5mg; Fiber: 2.5g; Protein: 16.1g

Slow Cooker Chickpea and Veggie Curry

Yield: 6 servings, Prep time: 10 minutes, Cook time: 3 hours

ALLERGEN-FRIENDLY, DAIRY-FREE, QUICK PREP, VEGAN/VEGETARIAN

Filling and flavorful best describe this Slow Cooker Chickpea and Veggie Curry. Serve this aromatic dish over cauliflower rice for a complete and hearty veggie-loaded meal.

1 (15.5-ounce) can chickpeas, drained and rinsed

2 cups cauliflower florets

1 cup Yukon gold potatoes, diced (about 3 small potatoes)

2 large carrots, sliced into rounds

1 bell pepper, chopped

1 (14.5-ounce) can diced tomatoes, with their juices

1 cup full-fat coconut milk

½ cup Basic Homemade Broth (page 163)

2 tablespoons curry powder

1 teaspoon garam masala

1 teaspoon kosher salt

Cauliflower rice, steamed or sautéed

Fresh cilantro (optional)

1. Put the chickpeas, cauliflower, potatoes, carrots, pepper, diced tomatoes and their juices, coconut milk, broth, curry powder, garam masala, and salt in a slow cooker and stir to combine.

2. Cook on high for 3 to 4 hours or on low for 6 to 7 hours.

3. Serve over cauliflower rice and top with chopped fresh cilantro (if using).

VARIATION TIP: For a spicier curry, add red pepper flakes before serving.

PER SERVING: Total calories: 205; Total fat: 8.7g; Saturated fat: 6.3g; Carbohydrates: 26g; Sodium: 599.7mg; Fiber: 7.1g; Protein: 6.7g

Tuscan Tomato–White Bean Bisque

Yield: 8 servings, Prep time: 10 minutes, Cook time: 20 minutes

30 MINUTES OR LESS, ALLERGEN-FRIENDLY, DAIRY-FREE, NUT-FREE, VEGAN/VEGETARIAN

You can still enjoy a creamy, comforting bisque-style soup without the dairy and gluten. Tuscan-inspired ingredients are simmered and blended to create a delicious silky tomato soup to enjoy with a side salad.

1 tablespoon extra-virgin olive oil

2 carrots, peeled and diced

2 stalks celery, diced

1 small onion, chopped

4 cloves garlic, minced

1 (28-ounce) can whole tomatoes

1 (15.5-ounce) can white cannellini beans, drained and rinsed

2 cups Basic Homemade Broth (page 163)

2 teaspoons dried rosemary

1 teaspoon sea salt

⅛ teaspoon red pepper flakes (optional)

1. In a large soup pot over medium-high heat, warm the olive oil. Add the carrots, celery, and onion. Cook for 5 minutes, stirring often, until the vegetables begin to soften.

2. Add the garlic, tomatoes, beans, broth, rosemary, and salt and bring to a boil. Use a wooden spoon to break up the tomatoes. Reduce the heat, cover, and simmer for 15 minutes.

3. Use an immersion blender to purée the soup, or carefully blend the soup in batches in a blender. If using a blender, cover the top with a towel to prevent spattering. Add red pepper flakes, if desired. Serve warm.

INGREDIENT TIP: Great northern beans and cannellini beans can be used interchangeably in most recipes.

PER SERVING: Total calories: 98; Total fat: 2g; Saturated fat: 0.3g; Carbohydrates: 16.7g; Sodium: 561.2mg; Fiber: 4.1g; Protein: 4.3g

Roasted Sweet Potato and Black Bean Farro Salad

Yield: 6 servings, Prep time: 10 minutes, Cook time: 30 minutes
ALLERGEN-FRIENDLY, DAIRY-FREE, NUT-FREE, VEGAN/VEGETARIAN

Farro, an underutilized but tasty and nutritious whole-grain option, is deliciously nutty and high in protein and fiber. In this salad, we'll pair farro with sweet potatoes, black beans, and a refreshing citrus dressing for a satisfying vegetarian meal.

3 tablespoons extra-virgin olive oil, divided, plus more to coat the pan

2 sweet potatoes, peeled and cut into ½-inch pieces

2 teaspoons sea salt, divided

1 teaspoon freshly ground black pepper, divided

2 cups cooked farro

1 (15.5-ounce) can low-sodium black beans, drained and rinsed

1 yellow bell pepper, diced

2 scallions, sliced

Juice of 1 lemon (about 2 tablespoons)

2 tablespoons chopped fresh parsley

1. Preheat the oven to 375°F. Grease a large rimmed baking sheet with olive oil and lay the sweet potatoes on the pan. Pour 1 tablespoon of olive oil, 1 teaspoon of salt, and ½ teaspoon of pepper over the potatoes and toss to coat.

2. Roast the sweet potatoes for 20 minutes, until tender and slightly browned. Remove from the oven and let cool.

3. In a large bowl, combine the cooked farro, potatoes, beans, bell pepper, and scallions.

4. Add the remaining 2 tablespoons of olive oil, 1 teaspoon of salt, ½ teaspoon of pepper, lemon juice, and parsley, and toss all ingredients to combine.

5. Serve immediately or refrigerate until ready to eat.

INGREDIENT TIP: Any color bell pepper can be used in this recipe.

PER SERVING: Total calories: 250; Total fat: 7.9g Saturated fat: 1g; Carbohydrates: 42.8g; Sodium: 783mg; Fiber: 7.2g; Protein: 8g

Taco Stuffed Peppers with Quinoa

Yield: 4 servings, Prep time: 10 minutes, Cook time: 35 minutes

ALLERGEN-FRIENDLY, DAIRY-FREE, NUT-FREE, QUICK PREP, VEGAN/VEGETARIAN

The classic stuffed pepper can be made so many ways. This meatless version features a Mexican flair and uses protein-rich quinoa in place of white rice, but it's still reminiscent of a traditional recipe. Make this family-friendly dish ahead and freeze it for future meals.

4 large bell peppers, any color

1 tablespoon extra-virgin olive oil

1 small yellow onion, diced

1 (14.5-ounce) can diced tomatoes

1 (4-ounce) can green chiles

2½ cups cooked quinoa

2 tablespoons Taco and Fajita Seasoning Blend (page 165)

1 teaspoon sea salt

1 (8-ounce) can unsalted tomato sauce

1. Preheat the oven to 350°F.

2. Cut the tops off the bell peppers. Remove the stems and chop the tops. Set aside.

3. In a large sauté pan or skillet over medium heat, warm the oil. Add the chopped peppers and onion. Cook for 5 minutes, stirring occasionally, until softened. Remove from the heat.

4. Add the diced tomatoes, green chiles, cooked quinoa, seasoning blend, and salt. Stir well to combine.

5. Place the bell peppers in a casserole dish and stuff with the quinoa mixture. Top each pepper with a spoonful of tomato sauce. Pour the remaining sauce into the bottom of the casserole dish.

6. Cover with foil and bake for 25 to 30 minutes, until the peppers are tender.

VARIATION TIP: Remove the foil in the last 5 minutes of cooking and top the peppers with shredded cheese for a decadent twist.

PER SERVING: Total calories: 278; Total fat: 6.5g; Saturated fat: 0.6g; Carbohydrates: 49.8g; Sodium: 1,044mg; Fiber: 9.5g; Protein: 8.6g

Easy Enchilada Quinoa Skillet

Yield: 6 cups, Prep time: 10 minutes, Cook time: 25 minutes
ALLERGEN-FREE, DAIRY-FREE, ONE-POT, VEGETARIAN

Quick prep, made in one pot, and totally family-friendly, this dish is perfect for busy nights. Make it your own by adding toppings.

1 tablespoon extra-virgin olive oil

1 small onion, diced

1 green bell pepper, diced

1 cup uncooked quinoa

1 (14.5-ounce) can fire-roasted tomatoes

1 (15.5-ounce) can low-sodium black beans, drained and rinsed

1 cup Basic Homemade Broth (page 163)

1 tablespoon Taco and Fajita Seasoning Blend (page 165)

1 teaspoon sea salt

1 cup spinach leaves

2 teaspoons freshly squeezed lime juice

Avocado, peeled, pitted, and diced, for topping (optional)

¼ cup shredded cheddar cheese, for topping (optional)

Diced tomatoes, for topping (optional)

Diced scallions, for topping (optional)

1. In a large deep sauté pan or skillet over medium heat, warm the oil. Add the onion and green pepper, and cook for 3 minutes, stirring occasionally.

2. Add the quinoa, tomatoes, beans, broth, seasoning blend, and salt. Bring to a boil, reduce the heat, cover, and simmer for 20 minutes, or until the quinoa is completely cooked.

3. In the last few minutes of cooking, uncover the pot and stir in the spinach leaves and lime juice.

4. Top with your favorite toppings such as diced avocados, shredded cheese, tomatoes, and scallions (if using).

VARIATION TIP: For a version with meat, stir in 8 ounces of cooked chicken, pork, or shrimp at step 3.

PER SERVING: Total calories: 235; Total fat: 4.3g; Saturated fat: 0.3g; Carbohydrates: 40.1g; Sodium: 695mg; Fiber: 6.8g; Protein: 9.3g

Veggie-Loaded Lentil Chili

Yield: 8 cups, Prep time: 10 minutes, Cook time: 4 hours

ALLERGEN-FRIENDLY, DAIRY-FREE, NUT-FREE, ONE-POT, VEGAN/VEGETARIAN

I love the endless possible combinations that I can make with chili. In this version, lentils and vegetables replace the meat for a nutritious plant-based, one-pot meal. Add some healthy fat to your bowl by topping this chili with diced avocado and finishing it with a sprinkle of fresh cilantro, if desired.

1 large green bell pepper, diced

1 small yellow onion, diced

1 cup frozen corn kernels

1 cup dried lentils, rinsed and sorted to remove debris

1 (15.5-ounce) can low-sodium black beans, drained and rinsed

½ cup diced carrots

½ cup diced zucchini

3½ cups Basic Homemade Broth (page 163)

2 cups crushed tomatoes

2 tablespoons Chili Seasoning Blend (page 164)

1. Combine the bell pepper, onion, corn, lentils, beans, carrots, zucchini, broth, tomatoes, and seasoning blend in a slow cooker. Stir well.

2. Cook on high for 4 to 5 hours or on low for 7 to 8 hours.

3. Serve warm.

SUBSTITUTION TIP: If you're not concerned with keeping this vegetarian, feel free to substitute chicken stock for the vegetable broth (see Variation tip, page 163).

PER SERVING: Total calories: 143; Total fat: 0.7g; Saturated fat: 0.1g; Carbohydrates: 31.3g; Sodium: 234.6mg; Fiber: 10.3g; Protein: 9.9g

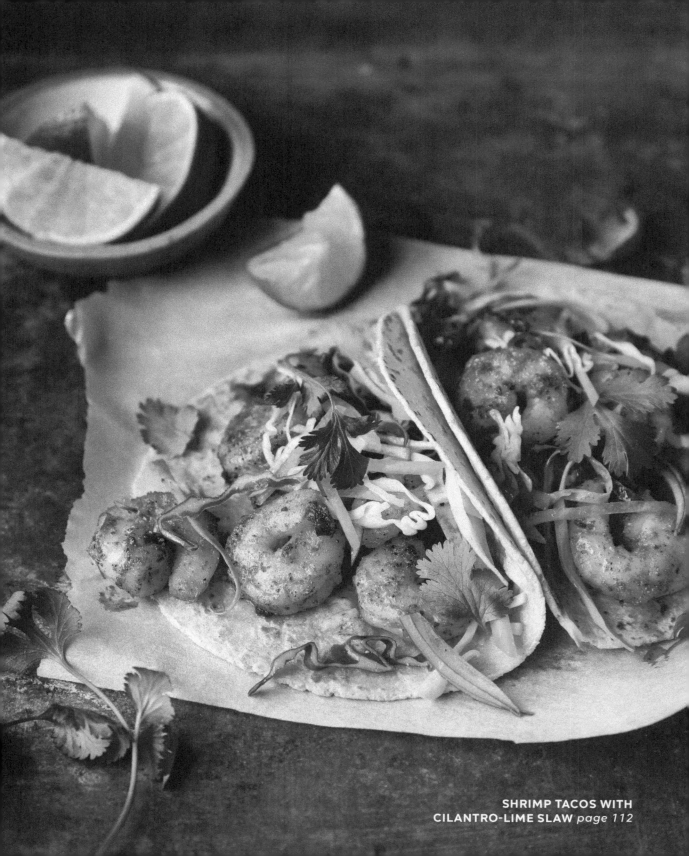

SHRIMP TACOS WITH
CILANTRO-LIME SLAW *page 112*

CHAPTER SEVEN

POULTRY AND SEAFOOD MAINS

Cashew Chicken Skillet

Yield: 4 servings, Prep time: 10 minutes, Cook time: 10 minutes

5 INGREDIENTS OR LESS, 30 MINUTES OR LESS, DAIRY-FREE, ONE-POT, QUICK PREP

You can easily make your favorite take-out dishes at home without sacrificing flavor. Cooking at home gives you the power to customize which ingredients go into your dishes, while also cutting your budget some slack. Enjoy this dish on its own or with a serving of brown rice or cauliflower rice.

1 tablespoon avocado oil or extra-virgin olive oil

1 pound boneless, skinless chicken breast, cut into 1-inch pieces

1 (12-ounce) bag frozen stir-fry vegetables (no sauce added)

½ cup unsalted roasted cashews

½ cup Stir-Fry Sauce (page 157)

1. In a large sauté pan or skillet over medium-high heat, warm the oil. Add the chicken and sauté for 3 to 4 minutes, until the chicken begins to brown.

2. Add the vegetables and continue to cook, stirring often, for another 3 to 4 minutes, until the vegetables begin to soften and the chicken is cooked through.

3. Add the cashews and sauce and stir until the sauce begins to thicken, 1 to 2 minutes. Serve hot.

INGREDIENT TIP: Frozen stir-fry vegetables are convenient in a pinch, but feel free to use fresh vegetables in this recipe. Other delicious add-ins include water chestnuts, bamboo shoots, and baby corn—just add them to the skillet at step 2.

PER SERVING: Total calories: 313; Total fat: 15.2g; Saturated fat: 2.7g; Carbohydrates: 19.2g; Sodium: 681mg; Fiber: 2.6g; Protein: 29.6g

Slow Cooker Chicken Tikka Masala

Yield: 6 servings, Prep time: 10 minutes, Cook time: 3 hours
ALLERGEN-FREE, DAIRY-FREE, NUT-FREE

If you've never made tikka masala, broaden your culinary horizons with this rich, flavorful, and slightly spicy dish. Enjoy this aromatic recipe over rice or cauliflower rice. Try adding some frozen green peas in the last hour of cooking time to add a boost of fiber and antioxidants.

1 small yellow onion, chopped

½ large yellow bell pepper, chopped

3 cloves garlic, minced

2 teaspoons garam masala

1½ teaspoons sea salt

1 teaspoon grated fresh ginger

1 teaspoon cumin

1 teaspoon coriander

1 teaspoon turmeric

¼ teaspoon cayenne pepper

1 (14.5-ounce) can diced tomatoes

½ cup full-fat coconut milk

2 pounds boneless, skinless chicken breasts

Fresh cilantro, for garnish (optional)

1. In a slow cooker, combine the onion, bell pepper, garlic, garam masala, salt, ginger, cumin, coriander, turmeric, cayenne pepper, tomatoes, and coconut milk. Stir well.

2. Add the chicken breasts, pressing down slightly to coat with the sauce. Cook on high for 3 to 4 hours or on low for 6 to 8 hours.

3. Remove the chicken breasts and shred with two forks. Set aside.

4. Using an immersion blender or standard blender, carefully purée the sauce until smooth.

5. Return the chicken to the sauce and stir well to coat. Serve with a sprinkle of fresh chopped cilantro (if using).

INGREDIENT TIP: Garam masala is available in most grocery stores, but you can make your own by combining 2 tablespoons of cumin, 1½ tablespoons of coriander, 1½ teaspoons of cinnamon, 1 tablespoon of cardamom, 1 tablespoon of freshly ground black pepper, ½ teaspoon of cloves, and ½ teaspoon of nutmeg.

PER SERVING: Total calories: 213; Total fat: 7.2g; Saturated fat: 3.7g; Carbohydrates: 6g; Sodium: 957mg; Fiber: 1g; Protein: 32g

Chicken Parmesan Meatballs

Yield: 6 servings, Prep time: 10 minutes, Cook time: 20 minutes
30 MINUTES OR LESS

These delectable meatballs are a lightened-up version of classic chicken Parmesan, big on flavor but not heavy on calories—and super easy to boot. Enjoy them served over zucchini noodles or alongside a green salad.

1 pound ground chicken

½ cup almond or oat flour (see Ingredient tip, page 72)

1 large egg, beaten

⅓ cup grated Parmesan cheese, plus more for garnish

1 tablespoon chopped fresh basil, plus more for garnish

½ teaspoon garlic powder

4 cups Marinara Sauce (page 152)

1. Preheat the oven to 425°F. Line a large rimmed baking sheet with parchment paper.

2. In a large bowl, combine the ground chicken, flour, egg, Parmesan, basil, and garlic powder. Mix well to incorporate all the ingredients.

3. Form the mixture into small, 1-inch meatballs and place on the baking sheet. Bake for 10 minutes, until the chicken is cooked through.

4. Meanwhile, in a large, deep sauté pan or skillet over medium heat, warm the marinara sauce.

5. Add the cooked meatballs to the sauce. Let the meatballs simmer in the sauce for 5 to 10 minutes. Serve warm, topped with additional Parmesan cheese and chopped basil, if desired.

SUBSTITUTION TIP: Make this dairy-free by substituting nutritional yeast for the Parmesan.

PER SERVING (5 MEATBALLS): Total calories: 260; Total fat: 15.9g; Saturated fat: 3.8g; Carbohydrates: 9.3g; Sodium: 543mg; Fiber: 2.4g; Protein: 24g

Citrus-Herb Roasted Whole Chicken with Quick Gravy

Yield: 6 servings, Prep time: 15 minutes, Cook time: 1½ hours

ALLERGEN-FRIENDLY, DAIRY-FREE, NUT-FREE

On a cold day, there's nothing better than a warm, comforting meal. Whip up the Creamy Cauliflower-Potato Mash (page 141) and your choice of vegetable to accompany the chicken.

For the chicken

1 (3- to 4-pound) whole chicken

1 lemon, cut into quarters

2 cloves garlic, peeled

¼ cup fresh parsley leaves, chopped

1 tablespoon kosher salt

1 tablespoon Poultry Seasoning Blend (page 164)

For the gravy

1 tablespoon arrowroot powder

2 tablespoons water

½ cup Basic Homemade Broth/Stock (page 163)

Sea salt

Freshly ground black pepper

To make the chicken

1. Preheat the oven to 325°F.

2. Rinse the chicken and pat the skin dry. Stuff the lemon quarters, garlic, and parsley leaves inside the chicken. Tie the legs together with kitchen twine and place in a roasting pan, breast-side up.

3. Sprinkle the surface of the chicken with the salt and poultry seasoning. Rub the seasoning into the skin.

4. Bake for about 20 minutes per pound, or until the internal temperature reaches 165°F in the thigh or thickest part of the chicken and the juices run clear.

5. Remove from the oven and let the chicken rest for 10 to 15 minutes, then transfer to a cutting board or serving platter. Reserve the pan juices.

To make the gravy

1. Strain the pan juices of any large pieces. Add the juices to a small pan and bring to a low simmer.

2. In a small dish, whisk together the arrowroot powder and water. Slowly add to the pan juices, whisking constantly until completely combined.

3. Continue to stir the gravy until it thickens, 1 to 2 minutes. If the gravy is too thick, add small amounts of broth until it reaches the desired consistency. Season with salt and pepper to taste.

INGREDIENT TIP: Reserve the chicken carcass from this recipe to make Basic Homemade Chicken Stock (Variation tip, page 163).

PER SERVING: Total calories: 186; Total fat: 7.6g; Saturated fat: 2.1g; Carbohydrates: 2.6g; Sodium: 1,265mg; Fiber: 0.2g; Protein: 25g

Turkey Sloppy Joes

Yield: 6 servings, Prep time: 10 minutes, Cook time: 20 minutes
30 MINUTES OR LESS, ALLERGEN-FRIENDLY, DAIRY-FREE, ONE-POT

Everyone in my family calls these sloppy joes a favorite. This version uses less sugar than traditional sloppy joes but is still reminiscent of Mom's classic recipe. Enjoy over a baked sweet potato for a fiber- and protein-rich meal.

1 tablespoon avocado oil or extra-virgin olive oil

2 pounds ground turkey

1 cup Clean Ketchup (page 151)

2 tablespoons apple cider vinegar

1 teaspoon honey

½ teaspoon garlic powder

½ teaspoon ground cloves

Sea salt

Freshly ground black pepper

1. In a large sauté pan or skillet over medium-high heat, warm the oil.

2. Add the turkey, breaking it up into small bits, and cook, stirring occasionally, for 5 to 6 minutes, or until fully browned.

3. Add the ketchup, vinegar, honey, garlic powder, cloves, salt, and pepper and stir well.

4. Bring the mixture to a low simmer and continue to cook until your desired consistency is reached, about 15 minutes. Serve warm.

SUBSTITUTION TIP: Ground beef or ground chicken can be used in place of the ground turkey.

PER SERVING: Total calories: 268; Total fat: 13g; Saturated fat: 3.7g; Carbohydrates: 8.3g; Sodium: 312mg; Fiber: 0.8g; Protein: 29.7g

Sheet-Pan Shrimp and Chicken Jambalaya

Yield: 6 servings, Prep time: 10 minutes, Cook time: 15 minutes

30 MINUTES OR LESS, DAIRY-FREE, ONE-PAN, QUICK PREP

My youngest daughter loves shrimp and requests this recipe regularly. She doesn't mind the little kick of Cajun spice, but if you're not a fan of spicy food, feel free to reduce or eliminate the cayenne pepper in the Cajun Seasoning Blend. Serve with white or cauliflower rice for a complete fuss-free meal, perfect for busy weeknights.

1½ pounds raw peeled and deveined shrimp

2 tablespoons extra-virgin olive oil, divided

2 tablespoons Cajun Seasoning Blend (page 164), divided

1 pound boneless, skinless chicken breast, cut into 1-inch cubes

2 large bell peppers, sliced (any color)

1 medium yellow onion, sliced

1. Preheat the oven to 400°F.

2. Rinse the shrimp and pat dry with paper towels. In a bowl, toss the shrimp with 1 tablespoon of oil and 1 tablespoon of Cajun Seasoning Blend. Set aside.

3. On a large rimmed baking sheet, add the chicken, peppers, and onion. Toss with the remaining 1 tablespoon of oil and 1 tablespoon of seasoning blend. Bake for 12 minutes, stirring once halfway through cooking.

4. Add the shrimp to the baking sheet and toss everything together. Bake for 3 to 4 minutes, until the chicken is cooked through and the shrimp are pink. Remove from the oven and serve warm.

VARIATION TIP: Change up the flavor profile by substituting a different seasoning blend, such as Taco and Fajita (page 165) or Mediterranean Seasoning Blend (page 164).

PER SERVING: Total calories: 257; Total fat: 8.5g; Saturated fat: 1.4g; Carbohydrates: 5.5g; Sodium: 285mg; Fiber: 1g; Protein: 39g

Shrimp Tacos
with Cilantro-Lime Slaw

Yield: 4 servings, Prep time: 15 minutes, plus 1 hour resting time, Cook time: 6 minutes

DAIRY-FREE, NUT-FREE

You'll love the ease of this recipe and its fresh, bold flavors. With quick-cooking shrimp and the help of a bagged coleslaw mix, this meal is ready in mere minutes after you've let the shrimp marinate. Serve these tacos in lettuce cups or corn tortillas with a dollop of Party Guacamole (page 158).

For the slaw

2 cups coleslaw mix

¼ cup thinly sliced red onion

3 tablespoons chopped fresh cilantro

2 tablespoons freshly squeezed lime juice

1½ tablespoons extra-virgin olive oil

¼ teaspoon sea salt

For the shrimp

1 pound raw peeled and deveined shrimp

2 tablespoons extra-virgin olive oil

2 tablespoons freshly squeezed lime juice

1 teaspoon minced garlic

1 tablespoon Taco and Fajita Seasoning Blend (page 165)

Lettuce cups or corn tortillas, for serving

1. For the slaw, in a bowl, pour in the coleslaw mix, red onion, and cilantro.

2. In a separate small bowl, whisk the lime juice, oil, and salt. Pour over the slaw and toss to combine. Cover and refrigerate to allow the flavors to meld.

3. Rinse the shrimp and pat dry with paper towels. Place the shrimp in a medium bowl.

4. In a small bowl, whisk together the olive oil, lime juice, garlic, and seasoning. Pour over the shrimp and toss to coat. Put in the refrigerator and let marinate for at least 15 minutes, up to 1 hour.

5. Heat a large sauté pan or skillet over medium-high heat. Pour the shrimp with the marinade into the pan and arrange the shrimp in a single layer.

6. Cook for about 2 minutes, until the edges of the shrimp begin to turn pink.

7. Flip the shrimp and cook for an additional 2 minutes, until the shrimp are pink and completely cooked through.

8. Serve the shrimp topped with the cilantro-lime slaw, in your choice of shell.

SUBSTITUTION TIP: Crispy Mahi Tenders (page 113) also make a great swap for the shrimp in these tacos.

PER SERVING: Total calories: 207; Total fat: 13.3g; Saturated fat: 1.8g; Carbohydrates: 4.8g; Sodium: 391.5mg; Fiber: 0.7g; Protein: 18.5g

Crispy Mahi Tenders

Yield: 4 servings, Prep time: 15 minutes, Cook time: 20 minutes

DAIRY-FREE

If you're trying to add more fish to your diet, mahi-mahi is a wonderful choice that is mild and kid-approved. These mahi tenders have a crispy coating even though they're baked instead of fried. Enjoy them with Cajun-Spiced Sweet Potato Fries (page 140) and a green salad.

Olive oil cooking spray

2 large eggs, beaten

½ cup almond flour

½ cup tapioca flour

1 teaspoon garlic powder

½ teaspoon sea salt

¼ teaspoon freshly ground black pepper

4 (6-ounce) mahi-mahi fillets, cut into 2-inch strips

Extra-virgin olive oil, for drizzling

1. Preheat the oven to 400°F. Spray a baking sheet with cooking spray.

2. Pour the beaten egg into a small bowl. In a medium bowl, whisk together the almond flour, tapioca flour, garlic powder, salt, and pepper.

3. Dip each mahi strip into the egg mixture and then the dry mixture, turning to coat evenly on all sides.

4. Place the strips on the baking sheet and drizzle with olive oil.

5. Bake for 15 to 18 minutes, until golden, flipping halfway through the baking time. Remove from the oven and serve warm.

SUBSTITUTION TIP: If you are nut-free, tapioca flour can be substituted for the almond flour.

PER SERVING: Total calories: 394; Total fat: 11.7g; Saturated fat: 1.3g; Carbohydrates: 19g; Sodium: 581.4mg; Fiber: 1.6g; Protein: 54.3g

Blackened Salmon with Cool Tomato-Cucumber Relish

Yield: 4 servings, Prep time: 15 minutes, Cook time: 10 minutes

30 MINUTES OR LESS, ALLERGEN-FRIENDLY, DAIRY-FREE, NUT-FREE, QUICK PREP

One of my husband's go-to meals at our favorite local restaurant is blackened salmon, so naturally I wanted to see if I could create the same thing at home. This recipe is definitely restaurant-worthy and so simple to make. The refreshing relish delivers a fresh and cooling balance to the rich and spicy salmon.

For the relish

⅓ cup finely diced English cucumber

½ cup seeded and finely diced tomatoes

1 teaspoon extra-virgin olive oil

1 teaspoon freshly squeezed lime juice

¼ teaspoon sea salt

For the blackening spice blend

1 tablespoon paprika

½ tablespoon garlic powder

½ tablespoon onion powder

½ tablespoon sea salt

1 teaspoon freshly ground black pepper

½ teaspoon cayenne pepper

½ teaspoon dried oregano

½ teaspoon thyme

For the salmon

4 (4- to 6-ounce) salmon fillets

2 tablespoons extra-virgin olive oil

To make the relish

In a small bowl, combine the cucumber, tomato, olive oil, lime juice, and salt. Toss to coat and refrigerate until ready to serve.

To make the blackening spice blend

In a small bowl, combine the paprika, garlic powder, onion powder, salt, black pepper, cayenne pepper, oregano, and thyme. Stir well and pour onto a large plate.

To make the salmon

1. Press the flesh side of each salmon fillet into the seasoning mixture, coating the salmon evenly.

2. In a large sauté pan or skillet over medium heat, warm the oil.

3. Place the salmon fillets, seasoned-side down, in the heated skillet. Cook for about 3 minutes, without disturbing the fillet. Flip and cook on the other side for an additional 2 to 3 minutes, or until the fish is cooked through and flakes easily with a fork.

4. Serve the salmon topped with the relish.

INGREDIENT TIP: Feel free to use either skin-on or skinless salmon fillets. For skinless, coat both sides of the salmon with the seasoning blend.

PER SERVING: Total calories: 256; Total fat: 11.5g; Saturated fat: 2g; Carbohydrates: 4.4g; Sodium: 1,223.6mg; Fiber: 1.5g; Protein: 35.5g

Garlic-Herb Salmon with Potato and Asparagus en Papillote

Yield: 4 servings, Prep time: 10 minutes, Cook time: 20 minutes

30 MINUTES OR LESS, QUICK PREP

The Mediterranean herbed butter that you can whip up in no time brings this dish to a new level. This recipe is easy but elegant enough to serve to company. Wrapping up the salmon and vegetables makes cleanup a breeze. *En papillote* means "in paper" in French, though you can also use foil.

¼ cup softened unsalted butter or ghee

2½ teaspoons Mediterranean Seasoning Blend, divided (page 164)

1½ teaspoons garlic powder

6 medium Yukon gold potatoes, sliced into thin rounds

1 pound asparagus, woody stems removed

4 (4- to 6-ounce) salmon fillets, skin removed

Fresh chopped parsley (optional)

1. Preheat the oven to 400°F. Set out 4 sheets of parchment paper and fold them in half.

2. In a small bowl, combine the softened butter, 1 teaspoon of Mediterranean seasoning, and garlic powder. Mix until well combined.

3. Divide the potatoes and asparagus evenly among the parchment pieces, placing the potatoes down the middle and the asparagus along the sides of the packet. Potato slices can overlap.

4. Place a salmon fillet on top of the potatoes in each parchment packet. Sprinkle the remaining Mediterranean seasoning over each foil packet.

5. Place a dollop of the herb butter on top of each salmon fillet.

6. Gather the tops and sides of the parchment together, folding the edges to seal, and forming tented envelopes. Place the envelopes on a large rimmed baking sheet.

7. Bake for 20 to 25 minutes, until the salmon is cooked through and flakes easily. Remove from the oven and serve immediately. If desired, top with fresh chopped parsley.

SUBSTITUTION TIP: You can swap out the potatoes and/or asparagus for sliced zucchini or bell peppers.

PER SERVING: Total calories: 461; Total fat: 14.7g; Saturated fat: 8g; Carbohydrates: 44.9g; Sodium: 206mg; Fiber: 5.5g; Protein: 42g

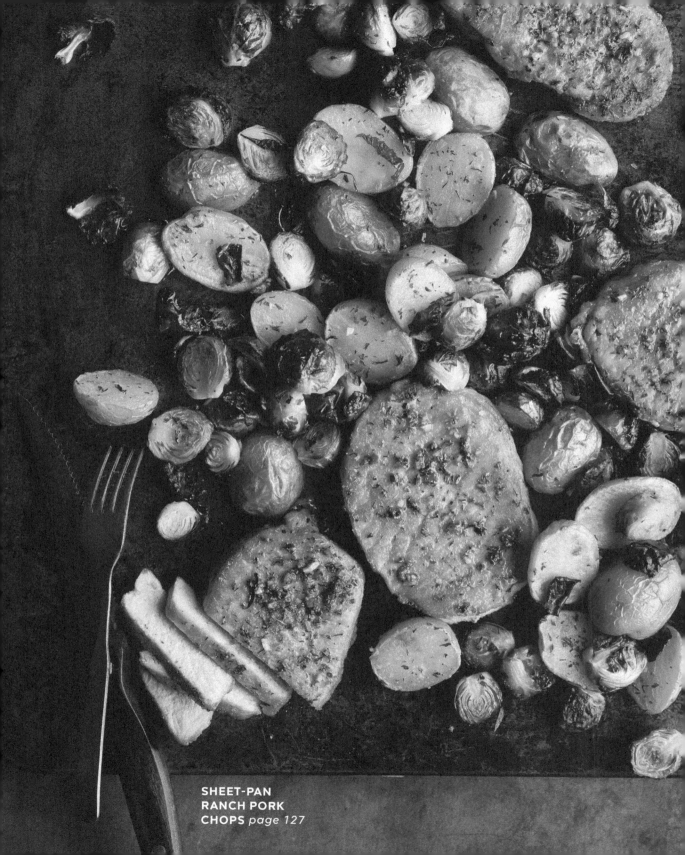

SHEET-PAN
RANCH PORK
CHOPS *page 127*

BEEF AND PORK MAINS

Mini Marinara Meatloaves

Yield: 12 mini meatloaves, Prep time: 10 minutes, Cook time: 20 minutes
5 INGREDIENTS OR LESS, 30 MINUTES OR LESS, DAIRY-FREE, QUICK PREP

Fiber-rich oats replace traditional bread crumbs in this meatloaf as a clean eating binding agent. Make these tasty mini meatloaves for dinner or add them to your weekly meal prep for a convenient make-ahead lunch option. This recipe can easily be doubled and frozen for future use.

Olive oil cooking spray

1½ pounds ground beef

½ cup whole rolled oats

⅔ cup Marinara Sauce (page 152), divided

1½ teaspoons Italian Seasoning Blend (page 164)

1 large egg

1 teaspoon sea salt

1. Preheat the oven to 350°F. Prepare a 12-cup muffin tin with cooking spray.

2. In a large bowl, combine the ground beef, oats, ⅓ cup of marinara, Italian seasoning, egg, and salt, and mix gently with your hands. Do not overmix.

3. Divide the mixture into 12 even scoops, placing one in each muffin cup and flattening slightly. Spread a teaspoon of additional marinara sauce on top of each muffin.

4. Bake for 18 to 20 minutes, or until cooked through. Remove from the oven and let sit for 5 minutes so any extra juices can reabsorb.

VARIATION TIP: You can easily change the flavor profile of these mini meatloaves by swapping out the sauce and seasoning. Try using Fresh Salsa (page 150) and Taco Seasoning Blend (page 165).

PER SERVING: Total calories: 117; Total fat: 5.7g; Saturated fat: 2.1g; Carbohydrates: 2.9g; Sodium: 265mg; Fiber: 0.5g; Protein: 13g

Skillet Shepherd's Pie

Yield: 6 servings, Prep time: 10 minutes, Cook time: 35 minutes
NUT-FREE, ONE-POT, QUICK PREP

Don't bother with those frozen store-bought potpies, which are full of unhealthy additives and plenty of sodium. Instead, make your own easy one-skillet shepherd's pie that hits the spot. The savory beef and vegetable base gets topped with Creamy Cauliflower-Potato Mash for a nutritious meal that will leave everyone satisfied.

1 tablespoon extra-virgin olive oil

½ cup diced onion

¾ cup diced carrots

1 pound lean ground beef or sirloin

1 teaspoon minced garlic

2 tablespoons tomato paste

1½ cups Basic Homemade Beef Stock (see Variation tip, page 163)

1 tablespoon light soy sauce

1 cup frozen peas

1 recipe Creamy Cauliflower-Potato Mash (page 141)

2 tablespoons unsalted butter

1. In a large, oven-safe sauté pan or skillet over medium-high heat, warm the oil. Add the onion and carrots and cook, stirring occasionally, until soft, 3 to 4 minutes. Add the ground beef and cook, stirring occasionally, until completely browned, 4 to 5 minutes.

2. Stir in the garlic and tomato paste. Add the broth and soy sauce. Stir well.

3. Bring the mixture to a boil, then reduce the heat and simmer uncovered for 15 to 20 minutes, or until the sauce reduces and thickens. Stir in the frozen peas.

4. Spread the warm cauliflower-potato mash over the top of the beef mixture. Remove from the heat.

5. Cut the butter into small pieces and scatter over the topping. Place the skillet in the oven under the broiler for 2 to 3 minutes, until golden brown. Serve hot.

VARIATION TIP: Use mashed sweet potatoes in place of the Creamy Cauliflower-Potato Mash.

PER SERVING: Total calories: 425; Total fat: 19.3g; Saturated fat: 9.8g; Carbohydrates: 42.9g; Sodium: 747.3mg; Fiber: 4.6g; Protein: 22g

Olive-Feta Sliders with Tzatziki Sauce

Yield: 8 sliders, Prep time: 10 minutes, Cook time: 15 minutes

30 MINUTES OR LESS, NUT-FREE, QUICK PREP

These juicy mini burgers are packed with flavor and perfect for serving as a game-day party snack or just a fun dinner. Make a salad with the leftovers to be enjoyed the next day for lunch.

1 pound lean ground beef or sirloin

¼ cup chopped Kalamata olives

¼ cup crumbled feta cheese

1 tablespoon chopped fresh parsley

2 tablespoons extra-virgin olive oil, divided

Iceberg lettuce leaves

2 Roma tomatoes, sliced

1 cup Tzatziki Sauce (page 159)

1. Line a plate with paper towels. Set aside.

2. In a large bowl, mix the ground beef, olives, feta, and parsley. Form the mixture into 2-inch patties. Flatten the patties and use your thumb to make an indentation in the center of each patty.

3. In a large sauté pan or skillet over medium-high heat, warm 1 tablespoon of oil. Add half of the sliders to the pan and cook for 3 to 4 minutes per side, until they reach your desired doneness. Repeat with remaining olive oil and patties.

4. Transfer the sliders to the lined plate to drain off any excess fat. Place each slider on a lettuce leaf. Serve topped with tomato slices and tzatziki sauce.

SUBSTITUTION TIP: This recipe can be made with ground turkey, lamb, or chicken instead of beef.

PER SERVING: Total calories: 184; Total fat: 13.2g; Saturated fat: 4g; Carbohydrates: 3.4g; Sodium: 441.7mg; Fiber: 0.3g; Protein: 13.3g

Stovetop Flank Steak Fajitas

Yield: 4 servings, Prep time: 10 minutes, Cook time: 15 minutes

30 MINUTES OR LESS, ALLERGEN-FRIENDLY, DAIRY-FREE, NUT-FREE, QUICK PREP

You *can* have tasty fajitas at home without using those packets of taco seasoning, which contain all kinds of unnecessary, even harmful additives not meant for your healthy body. Beloved in our house, fajitas make great eats for a quick family dinner or even when you need to feed a crowd. Set up a "make your own fajita" bar and serve with Fresh Salsa (page 150) and Party Guacamole (page 158), in warmed corn tortillas or over greens.

2 tablespoons extra-virgin olive oil, divided

1 red bell pepper, cut into strips

1 green bell pepper, cut into strips

1 medium red onion, sliced

2 tablespoons Taco and Fajita Seasoning Blend (page 165), divided

1 pound flank steak, cut into very thin strips

1 tablespoon freshly squeezed lime juice, for garnish

1 tablespoon fresh chopped cilantro, for garnish

1. In a large cast iron skillet (see Cooking tip) over medium-high heat, warm the oil. Add the bell peppers, onion, and 1 tablespoon of seasoning. Cook, stirring often, for 7 to 8 minutes, until the vegetables are soft.

2. Add the steak to the skillet, along with the remaining 1 tablespoon of seasoning. Cook, stirring occasionally, for 3 to 4 minutes for medium-rare steak, or longer to your desired doneness.

3. Sprinkle the steaks with the lime juice and cilantro. Serve immediately.

COOKING TIP: A large cast iron skillet works best for cooking fajitas on the stovetop and for getting a nice char on the peppers and onions. In the absence of a cast iron skillet, any large skillet will work.

PER SERVING: Total calories: 270 Total fat: 14.2g Saturated fat: 1g Carbohydrates: 9.3g Sodium: 315mg Fiber: 1.6g Protein: 25g

Sunday Pot Roast with Root Vegetables

Yield: 6 servings, Prep time: 10 minutes, Cook time: 3½ hours

ALLERGEN-FRIENDLY, DAIRY-FREE, NUT-FREE

Who doesn't love a wholesome family meal that is relatively hands-off and leaves the house smelling amazing? This Sunday Pot Roast with Root Vegetables fits the bill perfectly and makes for fantastic leftovers—if there are any.

1 tablespoon extra-virgin olive oil or avocado oil

1 (2- to 3-pound) boneless beef chuck roast

½ cup no-salt-added tomato sauce

1 cup Basic Homemade Beef Stock (see Variation tip, page 163)

1 medium yellow onion, sliced

1 teaspoon kosher salt

2 bay leaves

1 pound small red potatoes

1 pound parsnips, peeled and cut into large chunks

2 large carrots, peeled and cut into large chunks

1. In a large Dutch oven over medium-high heat, warm the oil. Add the beef and brown on all sides, 2 to 3 minutes per side.

2. Meanwhile, in a medium bowl, whisk together the tomato sauce and stock until combined. Pour the liquid over the roast, and add the onion, salt, and bay leaves to the pot. Bring to a boil, then reduce the heat, cover, and simmer over low heat for 1½ hours.

3. Add the potatoes, parsnips, and carrots to the pot, cover, and continue cooking on low for 1 to 1½ hours, until the beef is fork-tender and pulls apart easily.

4. Remove the bay leaves and serve warm.

COOKING TIP: At step 2, after bringing the liquid to a boil, add the vegetables and transfer the pot to a preheated 275°F oven. Roast uncovered for about 3 hours, until the beef is fork-tender.

PER SERVING: Total calories: 411; Total fat: 13.3g; Saturated fat: 4g ;Carbohydrates: 30g; Sodium: 615mg; Fiber: 5.9g; Protein: 42g

Thai Peanut Pork Lettuce Cups

Yield: 4 servings, Prep time: 10 minutes, Cook time: 15 minutes

30 MINUTES OR LESS, DAIRY-FREE, QUICK PREP

Sneak more veggies into your meals by hiding them in ground meat mixtures. The creamy, nutty sauce perfectly complements the pork and crunchy veggies.

For the pork

1 tablespoon extra-virgin olive oil

8 ounces mushrooms, finely chopped

1 pound ground pork

2 scallions, sliced

2 teaspoons minced garlic

1 teaspoon grated ginger

For the sauce

3 tablespoons light soy sauce or coconut aminos

2 tablespoons natural peanut butter (no sugar added)

1 teaspoon sesame oil

1 teaspoon fish sauce

For the garnish

8 to 12 Bibb lettuce leaves

½ red bell pepper, thinly sliced

1 medium grated carrot

¼ cup chopped unsalted roasted peanuts

Chopped fresh cilantro

Cayenne pepper hot sauce (optional)

1. In a large sauté pan or skillet over medium-high heat, warm the olive oil. Add the mushrooms and cook, stirring occasionally, for 2 to 3 minutes, until they begin to soften.

2. Add the ground pork and continue to cook for 3 to 4 minutes, breaking up the pork into small crumbles.

3. Stir in the scallions, garlic, and ginger and cook for 2 minutes, stirring frequently.

4. To make the sauce, in a small bowl, combine the soy sauce, peanut butter, sesame oil, and fish sauce. Whisk until smooth.

5. Pour the sauce into the pan with the pork mixture and stir well, cooking for an additional 2 minutes, then remove from heat.

6. To serve, spoon ¼ cup of the meat mixture into each lettuce cup. Top with bell peppers, carrots, peanuts, cilantro, and hot sauce (if using).

INGREDIENT TIP: For a spicier version of these lettuce cups, add some red pepper flakes to the sauce.

PER SERVING: Total calories: 531; Total fat: 37.9g; Saturated fat: 10.7g; Carbohydrates: 12.2g; Sodium: 654.7mg; Fiber: 3.7g; Protein: 37.9g

Slow Cooker Barbecue Pulled Pork

Yield: 8 servings, Prep time: 10 minutes, Cook time: 4 hours

ALLERGEN-FRIENDLY, DAIRY-FREE, NUT-FREE, ONE-POT, QUICK PREP

The more you discover how easy it is to cook different kinds of foods at home, the less you'll want to shell out money for pre-made dishes. Although you can make it in fewer hours on the slow cooker's high setting, "low and slow" is the way to go for truly tender meat. We enjoy this flavorful pulled pork over baked sweet potatoes. It makes enough to feed a crowd.

2 teaspoons smoked paprika

1½ teaspoons garlic powder

1½ teaspoons freshly ground black pepper

1 teaspoon cayenne pepper (optional)

1 teaspoon thyme

1 teaspoon sea salt

1 (3- to 4-pound) pork shoulder

1 cup water or Basic Homemade Broth (page 163)

1. In a small bowl, combine the paprika, garlic powder, black pepper, cayenne pepper (if using), thyme, and salt and mix well.

2. Trim any large areas of excess fat from the pork shoulder. Coat the pork with the spice mix by rubbing it on all sides.

3. Place the pork in a slow cooker and add the water or broth around the pork. Cook on high for 4 to 5 hours or on low for 7 to 8 hours.

4. While still warm, shred the pork using two forks.

COOKING TIP: For crispy, carnitas-style pork, spread the finished pulled pork in a large roasting pan, drizzle with ½ cup of the cooking juices, and place under the broiler for a few minutes, until the pork becomes golden and begins to get crispy.

PER SERVING: Total calories: 396; Total fat: 23g; Saturated fat: 8.2g; Carbohydrates: 1g; Sodium: 419mg; Fiber: 0.4g; Protein: 43g

Sheet-Pan Ranch Pork Chops

Yield: 4 servings, Prep time: 10 minutes, Cook time: 25 minutes

5 INGREDIENTS OR LESS, ALLERGEN-FRIENDLY, DAIRY-FREE, NUT-FREE, QUICK PREP

Sheet-pan meals are so versatile and easy to customize. Pick a protein, some veggies, and some sort of flavor booster and you have a complete meal cooked in one pan. The trick to sheet-pan meals: Choose ingredients that will cook in relatively the same amount of time or that cook in stages. In this recipe, pork loin chops, potatoes, Brussels sprouts, and a homemade ranch seasoning are the perfect combo.

2 tablespoons extra-virgin olive oil

2 tablespoons Ranch Seasoning Blend (page 164)

4 (4- to 5-ounce) boneless pork loin chops

1 pound small Yukon gold potatoes, halved

1 pound Brussels sprouts, halved

1. Preheat oven to 375°F. Line a rimmed baking sheet with parchment paper and set aside.

2. In a small bowl, whisk together the oil and ranch seasoning.

3. Arrange the pork chops, potatoes, and Brussels sprouts on the lined baking sheet.

4. Pour the seasoning mixture over the pork and vegetables and turn to coat.

5. Bake for 20 to 25 minutes, until the pork is cooked through.

VARIATION TIP: Use hearty vegetables in this recipe, such as broccoli, carrots, or cauliflower.

PER SERVING: Total calories: 330; Total fat: 12.4g; Saturated fat: 3.1g; Carbohydrates: 28.5g; Sodium: 714mg; Fiber: 7g; Protein: 27g

Garlic-Ginger Pork and Broccoli Stir-Fry

Yield: 4 servings, Prep time: 10 minutes, Cook time: 20 minutes

30 MINUTES OR LESS, ALLERGEN-FRIENDLY, DAIRY-FREE, NUT-FREE, ONE-PAN, QUICK PREP

You can make your own take-out-rivaling stir-fry at home for a fraction of the sodium and fat—not to mention the cost. Enjoy this tasty dish on its own or serve with cauliflower rice for a complete meal.

1½ tablespoons extra-virgin olive oil, divided

1 pound boneless pork loin chops, cut into thin strips

8 ounces sliced mushrooms

2 cups broccoli florets

1 teaspoon minced garlic

1 teaspoon grated ginger

½ cup Stir-Fry Sauce (page 157)

1. In a large sauté pan or skillet over medium-high heat, warm 1 tablespoon of oil. Add the pork and cook, stirring and turning often, until no longer pink, about 5 minutes. Remove the pork from the pan and set aside.

2. In the same skillet, add the remaining ½ tablespoon of oil and mushrooms. Cook for 2 to 3 minutes, stirring often, until the mushrooms are softened.

3. Add the broccoli to the skillet and cook for 2 to 3 minutes, until bright green.

4. Stir in the garlic and ginger, and cook for 1 minute, stirring frequently.

5. Add the stir-fry sauce and stir to combine. Cook for 2 to 3 minutes, stirring occasionally, until the sauce has thickened slightly.

6. Add the pork back to the pan and stir to combine. Serve immediately.

VARIATION TIP: Add red bell pepper strips, sliced carrots, and water chestnuts with the mushrooms.

PER SERVING: Total calories: 234; Total fat: 11.2g; Saturated fat: 2.9g; Carbohydrates: 8.8g; Sodium: 1,086mg; Fiber: 0.8g; Protein: 24g

Rosemary-Dijon Pork Tenderloin with Roasted Potatoes and Carrots

Yield: 4 servings, Prep time: 30 minutes, Cook time: 25 minutes

ALLERGEN-FRIENDLY, DAIRY-FREE, NUT-FREE, QUICK PREP

I originally created my Rosemary and Dijon Marinade for use with turkey tenderloin but realized quickly that it is an all-around winner with any kind of protein, especially pork and chicken. I love the rustic flavors and simplicity of this recipe and my kids and husband always go back for seconds. If you're new to pork tenderloins, they usually come packaged two to a pack.

2 (1-pound) pork tenderloins

1 recipe Rosemary and Dijon Marinade (page 162)

1 pound baby red potatoes, halved

1 pound baby carrots

1 tablespoon extra-virgin olive oil

1 teaspoon kosher salt

½ teaspoon freshly ground black pepper

1. Preheat the oven to 375°F.

2. Place the pork tenderloins in a large baking dish. Pour the marinade over top and turn to coat. Cover and refrigerate for at least 30 minutes.

3. On a large rimmed baking sheet, toss the potatoes, carrots, oil, salt, and pepper.

4. Push the vegetables to the sides of the baking sheet, and arrange the pork tenderloin in the middle.

5. Bake for 20 to 25 minutes, until the pork is cooked through.

COOKING TIP: If you prefer, the pork tenderloins can be grilled rather than baked. Wrap up the veggies in foil and cook them on the grill, too.

PER SERVING: Total calories: 693; Total fat: 29.3g; Saturated fat: 6.4g; Carbohydrates: 32g; Sodium: 1,461mg; Fiber: 5.5g; Protein: 71g

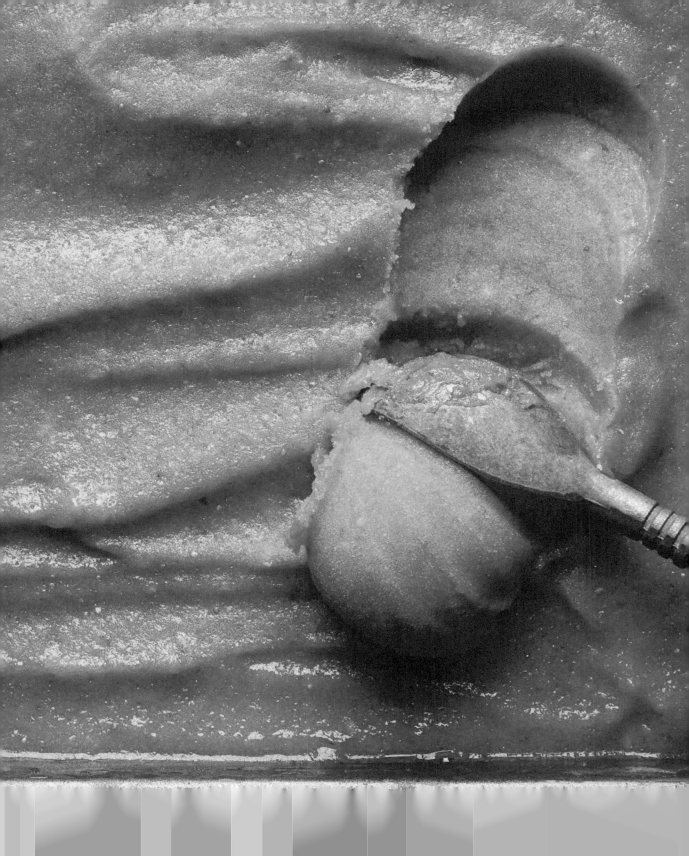

CHAPTER NINE

SNACKS, SIDES, AND DESSERTS

Nutty Cranberry Oat Bites

Yield: 24 bites, Prep time: 10 minutes, plus 30 minutes chilling time
DAIRY-FREE, VEGETARIAN

Snacks are an important piece of the clean eating puzzle. With so many tempting store-bought options out there, you'll want to build your arsenal of really great snack recipes. These tasty no-cook bites are the perfect on-the-go snack and are super kid-friendly. I love to have these protein-packed treats on hand for a healthy lunch box snack or post-workout energy booster.

1 cup whole rolled oats

¾ cup ground walnuts (see Ingredient tip)

½ cup crunchy natural peanut butter (no sugar added)

¼ cup honey

2 tablespoons ground flaxseed

½ teaspoon cinnamon

½ teaspoon vanilla extract

¼ cup dried, no-sugar-added cranberries

1. Line a baking sheet with wax paper and set aside.

2. In a bowl, combine the oats, ground walnuts, peanut butter, honey, flaxseed, cinnamon, and vanilla. Mix until everything is well incorporated. Stir in the cranberries.

3. Form the dough into 1-inch balls and place on the prepared baking sheet. Chill in the refrigerator or freezer until set, at least 30 minutes.

4. Store in an airtight container in the refrigerator for up to 1 week.

INGREDIENT TIP: Grind the walnuts in a food processor, pulsing until they reach a crumb-like consistency. You can also use ground pecans, hazelnuts, or macadamia nuts.

PER SERVING: Total calories: 82; Total fat: 5g; Saturated fat: 0.6g; Carbohydrates: 7.7g; Sodium: 20mg; Fiber: 1g; Protein: 2g

Crispy Ranch Chickpeas

Yield: 3½ cups, Prep time: 10 minutes, Cook time: 45 minutes

5 INGREDIENTS OR LESS, ALLERGEN-FRIENDLY, DAIRY-FREE, NUT-FREE, QUICK PREP, VEGAN/VEGETARIAN

Chickpeas are a nutrient-dense alternative to the unhealthy crunchy snacks found in the chip aisle. To achieve extra-crispy chickpeas, be sure to dry them completely before baking and store them uncovered, as sealing them in a container will create moisture and the chickpeas will lose their crispiness. But really, they are best enjoyed right away!

2 (15.5-ounce) cans chickpeas, drained and rinsed

½ tablespoon avocado oil or extra-virgin olive oil

1½ tablespoons Ranch Seasoning Blend (page 164)

1 teaspoon sea salt

1. Preheat the oven to 375°F.

2. Using paper towels or a large, clean dish towel, completely dry the chickpeas.

3. Spread the dry chickpeas in a single layer on a large rimmed baking sheet. Bake for 10 minutes.

4. Remove the baking sheet from the oven and add the oil, tossing well. Bake for an additional 25 minutes, shaking the pan once or twice throughout.

5. Sprinkle the seasoning and salt over the chickpeas and toss well to combine. Let cool on the pan for at least 20 minutes to allow them to crisp up more.

SUBSTITUTION TIP: Any of the homemade seasoning blends from pages 164 and 165 can be used in place of the Ranch Seasoning Blend.

PER ½ CUP: Total calories: 134; Total fat: 2.9g; Saturated fat: 0.3g; Carbohydrates: 20.8g; Sodium: 376mg; Fiber: 5.7g; Protein: 6.6g

Baked Granola

Yield: 6 cups, Prep time: 5 minutes, Cook time: 25 minutes

30 MINUTES OR LESS, DAIRY-FREE, QUICK PREP, VEGETARIAN

Naturally sweetened and full of fiber and nutrients, homemade baked granola can be enjoyed as a snack on its own, with oatmeal (see Overnight Oats, page 70) or as a topping for fruit desserts. This basic recipe can be jazzed up with other delicious add-ins like nuts, coconut, and dried fruit. Make it your own with your favorite ingredients.

Olive oil cooking spray

4 cups whole rolled oats

1½ cups raw slivered almonds

¼ cup chia seeds

1½ teaspoons cinnamon

1 teaspoon sea salt

½ cup pure maple syrup or honey

½ cup melted unrefined coconut oil

1 teaspoon vanilla extract

½ cup unsweetened coconut flakes

1. Preheat the oven to 350°F. Prepare a large rimmed baking sheet with cooking spray.

2. In a large bowl, combine the oats, almonds, chia seeds, cinnamon, and salt. Mix well.

3. Drizzle the maple syrup, coconut oil, and vanilla over the oat mixture. Toss well to coat evenly.

4. Spread the mixture on the prepared baking sheet and bake for 20 to 25 minutes, stirring once halfway through cooking. In the last 5 minutes of baking, add the coconut flakes to the pan.

5. Let the granola sit and cool for at least 30 minutes. Break the granola into large chunks or smaller pieces if desired, and store in an airtight container at room temperature for up to 2 weeks.

INGREDIENT TIP: Dried fruit such as raisins or cranberries can be added to the granola after baking.

PER ½ CUP: Total calories: 329; Total fat: 20.5g; Saturated fat: 9.9g; Carbohydrates: 32.3g; Sodium: 196mg; Fiber: 6.5g; Protein: 7.4g

Quick Refrigerator Pickles

Yield: 1 (32-ounce) jar, Prep time: 5 minutes, plus 24 hours marinating time

5 INGREDIENTS OR LESS, ALLERGEN-FRIENDLY, DAIRY-FREE, NUT-FREE, QUICK PREP, VEGAN/VEGETARIAN

Enjoy this quick and easy snack when you're craving something crunchy and salty. I love to pair these super crunchy pickles with a healthy fat like olives when I need something to perk up my taste buds and tide me over to my next meal.

1 cup water

1 cup white vinegar

1 tablespoon kosher salt

2 cloves garlic, sliced

3 or 4 sprigs fresh dill

1 large English cucumber

1. In a quart-size Mason jar, pour in the water, vinegar, salt, garlic, and dill sprigs. Tighten the lid and shake to combine.

2. Slice the cucumber into spears or ¼-inch rounds. Add them to the water and vinegar mixture.

3. Seal the jar and refrigerate for at least 24 hours before serving. Store refrigerated for up to 7 to 10 days.

INGREDIENT TIP: Be sure to use English cucumbers or small pickling cucumbers for the best results. They don't contain the large seeds that a regular cucumber has, and they tend to be firmer, resulting in a crunchier pickle.

PER JAR: Total calories: 54; Total fat: 0g; Saturated fat: 0g; Carbohydrates: 11g; Sodium: 6,978mg; Fiber: 1.1g; Protein: 3.4g

Roasted Rosemary Mixed Nuts

Yield: 3 cups, Prep time: 10 minutes, Cook time: 40 minutes

5 INGREDIENTS OR LESS, DAIRY-FREE, QUICK PREP, VEGETARIAN

Nuts are a superfood in the sense that they are a natural source of protein and healthy fats. Enjoy a handful of these roasted spiced nuts as a convenient, portable snack or add them over the tops of salads for some crunch. I also love to pulse them in a food processor to make a "breading" for baked chicken and fish.

Olive oil cooking spray

1 cup raw cashews

1 cup raw almonds

1 cup raw pecans

1 egg white, beaten until frothy

2 teaspoons minced fresh rosemary

1½ teaspoons sea salt

1. Preheat the oven to 300°F. Line a large rimmed baking sheet with parchment paper. Spray lightly with olive oil cooking spray. Set aside.

2. Pour the cashews, almonds, and pecans into a large bowl with the egg white and toss well to combine.

3. In a small bowl, stir together the rosemary and salt. Sprinkle the mixture over the nuts and stir to coat evenly.

4. Spread the nuts in a single layer on the baking sheet. Bake for 40 minutes, stirring every 15 minutes, until lightly browned and crunchy. Store for up to 1 week in an airtight container in the refrigerator or at room temperature.

INGREDIENT TIP: Always look for the raw, unsalted nuts in the store. They shouldn't contain sugar, extra sodium, or other preservatives.

PER ½ CUP: Total calories: 394; Total fat: 35.2g; Saturated fat: 4.1g; Carbohydrates: 15.1g; Sodium: 594mg; Fiber: 5.3g; Protein: 11g

Crunchy Almond Broccoli Slaw

Yield: 6 servings, Prep time: 10 minutes

DAIRY-FREE, QUICK PREP, VEGAN/VEGETARIAN

If green salads are growing a little stale, try this crunchy broccoli slaw for a change of pace. Make it a complete meal by adding some shredded chicken or serve as a side dish alongside Slow Cooker Barbecue Pulled Pork (page 126) or another grilled meat.

1 (10-ounce) bag broccoli slaw

½ red bell pepper, thinly sliced

¼ cup matchstick carrots

¼ cup slivered almonds

¼ cup sunflower seeds

2 scallions, sliced

¼ cup Sesame-Ginger Dressing (page 154)

1 tablespoon sesame seeds (optional)

1. In a large bowl, combine the broccoli slaw, bell pepper, carrots, almonds, sunflower seeds, scallions, and dressing. Toss well to coat the salad with the dressing.

2. Sprinkle with sesame seeds (if using) and serve immediately, or cover and refrigerate until ready to eat (see Serving tip).

3. Salad will keep for up to 2 days in the refrigerator.

SERVING TIP: If prepping this salad more than a day in advance or for make-ahead lunches, keep the salad ingredients and dressing separate until ready to serve.

PER SERVING: Total calories: 125; Total fat: 7.8g; Saturated fat: 0.9g; Carbohydrates: 12.1g; Sodium: 194.8mg; Fiber: 3.6g; Protein: 3.8g

Baked Broccoli Fritters

Yield: 10 fritters, Prep time: 10 minutes, Cook time: 25 minutes

QUICK PREP, VEGETARIAN

Fritters are a fun and tasty way to get your veggies in—yes, these count as veggies! Serve along with supper or as an appetizer with a little Creamy Ranch Dressing (page 155) for dipping. To make this recipe dairy-free, substitute nutritional yeast for the Parmesan.

1 head broccoli, florets only

¼ cup finely diced yellow onion

1 large egg, beaten

½ cup cassava or almond flour

1 teaspoon lemon zest

½ teaspoon garlic powder

1 teaspoon sea salt

¼ cup grated Parmesan cheese

2 tablespoons extra-virgin olive oil

1. Preheat the oven to 400°F. Line a baking sheet with parchment paper.

2. Put the broccoli florets in a food processor and pulse until finely chopped. Pour into a large bowl.

3. Add the onion, egg, flour, lemon zest, garlic powder, salt, and Parmesan, and combine well to form a dough. Form 8 patties and place on the prepared baking sheet.

4. Drizzle patties with olive oil and bake for 25 to 30 minutes, flipping halfway through, until lightly browned on both sides.

COOKING TIP: To cook on the stovetop, heat the olive oil in a large sauté pan or skillet (instead of drizzling) and pan fry the patties for about 3 minutes per side, until browned.

PER SERVING: Total calories: 84; Total fat: 4.3g; Saturated fat: 1.1g; Carbohydrates: 9g; Sodium: 303mg; Fiber: 2.3g; Protein: 4g

Balsamic Roasted Vegetables

Yield: 6 servings, Prep time: 10 minutes, Cook time: 30 minutes

ALLERGEN-FRIENDLY, DAIRY-FREE, NUT-FREE, QUICK PREP, VEGAN/VEGETARIAN

Think you're not a vegetable fan? Try roasting your veggies. Roasting is a fuss-free way to cook vegetables and creates a sweet, mellow flavor on the inside while giving a little crisp to the outside. Pair these Balsamic Roasted Vegetables with Citrus-Herb Roasted Whole Chicken with Quick Gravy (page 109) or Crispy Mahi Tenders (page 113) for a meal bursting with flavor.

8 ounces Brussels sprouts, halved

1 red bell pepper, cut into chunks

½ red onion, cut into chunks

1 medium zucchini, cut into 1-inch chunks

2 cups cauliflower florets

3 tablespoons balsamic vinegar

2 tablespoons extra-virgin olive oil

2 teaspoons Italian Seasoning Blend (page 164), or store-bought Italian seasoning

1 teaspoon kosher salt

1. Preheat the oven to 400°F. Line a large rimmed baking sheet with parchment paper.

2. Spread the Brussels sprouts, bell pepper, red onion, zucchini, and cauliflower on the lined baking sheet.

3. In a small bowl, whisk together the balsamic vinegar, olive oil, Italian seasoning, and salt. Pour the liquid over the vegetables and toss to combine, then spread the vegetables back out in an even layer.

4. Roast for 25 to 30 minutes, until the vegetables are fork-tender and beginning to brown.

SUBSTITUTION TIP: Substitute broccoli, baby potatoes, or carrots for any of the vegetables in this recipe.

PER SERVING: Total calories: 84; Total fat: 5g; Saturated fat: 0.7g; Carbohydrates: 9.7g; Sodium: 413mg; Fiber: 3.4g; Protein: 3g

Cajun-Spiced Sweet Potato Fries

Yield: 4 servings, Prep time: 10 minutes, Cook time: 30 minutes

5 INGREDIENTS OR LESS, ALLERGEN-FRIENDLY, DAIRY-FREE, NUT-FREE, QUICK PREP, VEGAN/VEGETARIAN

Rich in the antioxidant beta-carotene, fiber, and many beneficial vitamins and minerals, sweet potatoes are a super versatile side dish. They are delicious roasted, added to chili or grain salads (see Roasted Sweet Potato and Black Bean Farro Salad, page 100), and in this case, cut into crispy fries. The Cajun spice in this recipe offers a spicy contrast to the sweetness of the fries.

2 large sweet potatoes

1½ tablespoons extra-virgin olive oil

2 tablespoons Cajun Seasoning Blend (page 164)

1. Preheat the oven to 425°F.

2. Cut the sweet potatoes into long, ½-inch-wide strips. Arrange on a large rimmed baking sheet.

3. Pour the oil over the fries and sprinkle with the seasoning, then toss well to coat.

4. Arrange in a single layer and bake for 25 to 30 minutes, flipping the fries once after 10 minutes. The fries are done when the edges begin to brown.

VARIATION TIP: For a milder version, reduce or omit the cayenne in the seasoning blend.

PER SERVING: Total calories: 126; Total fat: 5.3g; Saturated fat: 0.8g; Carbohydrates: 18.5g; Sodium: 830mg; Fiber: 3g; Protein: 2g

Creamy Cauliflower-Potato Mash

Yield: 8 servings, Prep time: 10 minutes, Cook time: 20 minutes

**5 INGREDIENTS OR LESS, 30 MINUTES OR LESS, ONE-POT,
QUICK PREP, VEGETARIAN**

If you haven't yet tried cauliflower as a substitute for potatoes and rice, start out with this hybrid recipe. You won't notice the cauliflower, but you'll enjoy all the benefits of this nutrient-dense vegetable. Serve with Sunday Pot Roast and Root Vegetables (page 124), Citrus-Herb Roasted Whole Chicken with Quick Gravy (page 109), or your favorite protein cooked your way.

5 medium russet potatoes, peeled and quartered

1 small head cauliflower, cut into chunks

3 tablespoons unsalted butter or ghee

1 teaspoon kosher salt

¼ cup coconut milk

Freshly ground black pepper

1. In a large pot, combine the potatoes and cauliflower, and cover with cold water. Bring to a boil over high heat.

2. Simmer uncovered for 15 minutes, or until the potatoes are fork-tender. Drain and return the potatoes and cauliflower to the pot.

3. Add the butter, salt, and coconut milk to the potatoes and cauliflower.

4. Mash with a potato masher, or use a hand mixer for a whipped potato consistency.

5. Season with salt and pepper.

INGREDIENT TIP: Brighten this dish by stirring in fresh chopped herbs like parsley, dill, or thyme.

PER SERVING: Total calories: 168; Total fat: 5.7g; Saturated fat: 3.8g; Carbohydrates: 26g; Sodium: 303mg; Fiber: 2g; Protein: 4g

Fudge Pops

Yield: 6 pops, Prep time: 10 minutes, plus 3 hours freezing time

**5 INGREDIENTS OR LESS, ALLERGEN-FRIENDLY, DAIRY-FREE,
QUICK PREP, VEGETARIAN**

Free of refined sugar and dairy, these creamy Fudge Pops can be enjoyed as a sweet snack on a hot day or anytime you are craving a cool, chocolatey treat. With only three ingredients, these pops are easy to whip up in no time, and any Popsicle mold shape will work well.

1 (13.5-ounce) can full-fat coconut milk

⅓ cup cocoa powder

¼ cup honey or maple syrup

1. In a blender or food processor, blend the milk, cocoa powder, and honey until smooth and creamy.

2. Pour into Popsicle molds and place in the freezer until frozen, 3 to 4 hours.

3. Run a little warm water over the outside of the molds to free the pops from their molds. Serve immediately.

VARIATION TIP: Add 2 tablespoons of natural peanut butter or almond butter for a chocolate-nut butter version.

PER SERVING: Total calories: 171; Total fat: 12.4g; Saturated fat: 10.4g; Carbohydrates: 16g Sodium: 18mg; Fiber: 1.6g; Protein: 2g

Apple Crisp

Yield: 6 servings, Prep time: 10 minutes, Cook time: 20 minutes

ALLERGEN-FRIENDLY, DAIRY-FREE, QUICK PREP, VEGAN/VEGETARIAN

Apple crisp makes your home smell amazing while it bakes—another great benefit of making your own from ingredients you select. A simple crumble topping provides the perfect crunchy contrast to the sweet, tender apples.

Olive oil cooking spray, for greasing the pan

4 cups thinly sliced apples

1½ teaspoons cinnamon, divided

1 cup whole rolled oats

½ cup finely chopped walnuts

1½ tablespoons coconut oil

2 tablespoons pure maple syrup

¼ teaspoon nutmeg

1. Preheat the oven to 350°F. Prepare a 9-inch pie plate with cooking spray.

2. Spread the apple slices in the prepared pie plate and sprinkle with ½ teaspoon of cinnamon.

3. In a separate bowl, combine the oats, walnuts, coconut oil, maple syrup, remaining 1 teaspoon of cinnamon, and nutmeg. Spread over top of the apples.

4. Bake for 30 to 35 minutes, until the apples are soft and topping is golden brown.

INGREDIENT TIP: To avoid using extra sugars in this dish, I like to use a sweeter variety of apple, like Gala, Honeycrisp, or Fuji.

PER SERVING: Total calories: 203; Total fat: 11.3g; Saturated fat: 3.6g; Carbohydrates: 25.5g; Sodium: 1mg; Fiber: 4.1g; Protein: 3.4g

Mango Soft Serve

Yield: 3 cups, Prep time: 5 minutes

**5 INGREDIENTS OR LESS, ALLERGEN-FRIENDLY, DAIRY-FREE,
NUT-FREE, QUICK PREP, VEGAN/VEGETARIAN**

No added sweeteners are necessary in this tropical-tasting creamy dessert. Just mango and bananas are blended to a soft-serve consistency, perfect for an after dinner sweet treat or quick snack.

2 cups frozen mango chunks, slightly thawed

2 bananas

1. Using a high-speed blender or food processor, blend the mangos and bananas until completely smooth. You may need to scrape down the sides several times or use a tamper to keep the mixture from seizing up.

2. Enjoy immediately. The soft serve can be set in the freezer, but it will take on an icier texture closer to sorbet once it is frozen.

COOKING TIP: A high-speed blender works best for puréeing frozen fruit and achieving a creamy texture.

PER CUP: Total calories: 130; Total fat: 0.6g; Saturated fat: 0.1g; Carbohydrates: 32g; Sodium: 1mg; Fiber: 3.4g; Protein: 1.5g

No-Bake Chocolate–Almond Butter Bars

Yield: 9 bars, Prep time: 10 minutes, Cook time: 1 hour

DAIRY-FREE, QUICK PREP, VEGETARIAN

Whip up these quick, no-bake bars for a convenient, energy-boosting treat. Cocoa, oats, and almond butter provide additional benefits like antioxidants, protein, and fiber, unlike most processed sweet treats, which tend to be devoid of any nutrients.

Olive oil cooking spray

¼ cup melted unrefined coconut oil

⅓ cup almond butter

⅓ cup honey

½ teaspoon vanilla extract

⅓ cup cocoa powder

¼ teaspoon sea salt

2¼ cups whole rolled oats

1. Prepare an 8-by-8-inch baking dish with cooking spray. Set aside.

2. In a large bowl, combine the melted coconut oil, almond butter, honey, and vanilla. Stir until completely mixed and smooth.

3. Stir in the cocoa powder and salt. Fold in the oats until completely combined.

4. Press the mixture into the prepared baking dish. Refrigerate for 1 hour, until completely set.

5. Once set, cut into bars and serve. If storing, keep in an airtight container in the refrigerator for up to 1 week.

VARIATION TIP: Make into bite-size pieces by rolling the mixture into 1-inch balls.

PER SERVING: Total calories: 230; Total fat: 13.3g; Saturated fat: 6g; Carbohydrates: 27.4g; Sodium: 66.8mg; Fiber: 4g; Protein: 4.5g

Quick Berry Sorbet

Yield: 4 cups, Prep time: 10 minutes, plus 30 minutes freezing time

5 INGREDIENTS OR LESS, ALLERGEN-FRIENDLY, DAIRY-FREE, NUT-FREE, QUICK PREP, VEGETARIAN

A sweet, light, and refreshing dessert is all yours, and you won't believe how easy it is to make. Use a mix of berries (raspberries, blueberries, etc.) or your preferred frozen fruit to customize this recipe to your taste.

4 cups frozen strawberries, slightly thawed

¼ cup honey

1. Put the semi-thawed strawberries into the bowl of a food processor or high-speed blender. Add the honey.

2. Process the mixture until smooth and creamy.

3. Pour the mixture into a freezer-safe, loaf-size pan and set in the freezer for at least 30 minutes, or until frozen.

4. Remove the sorbet when ready to eat and let stand for a few minutes until easy to scoop.

VARIATION TIP: Go with whatever's in season—for example, frozen sweet peaches offer another delicious option and they don't even require a sweetener.

PER CUP: Total calories: 116; Total fat: 0.2g; Saturated fat: 0g; Carbohydrates: 31.1g; Sodium: 3.8mg; Fiber: 3.1g; Protein: 0.7g

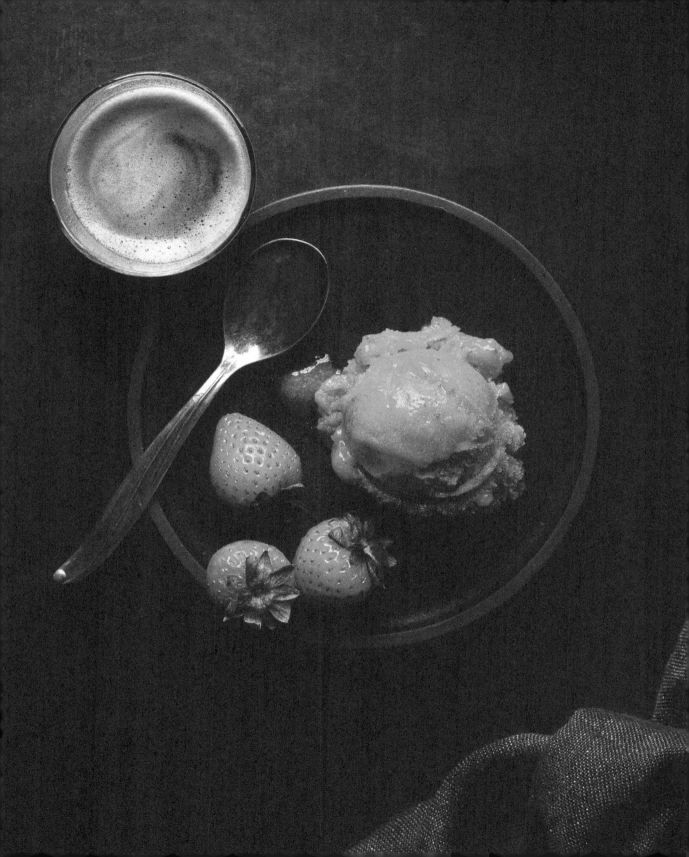

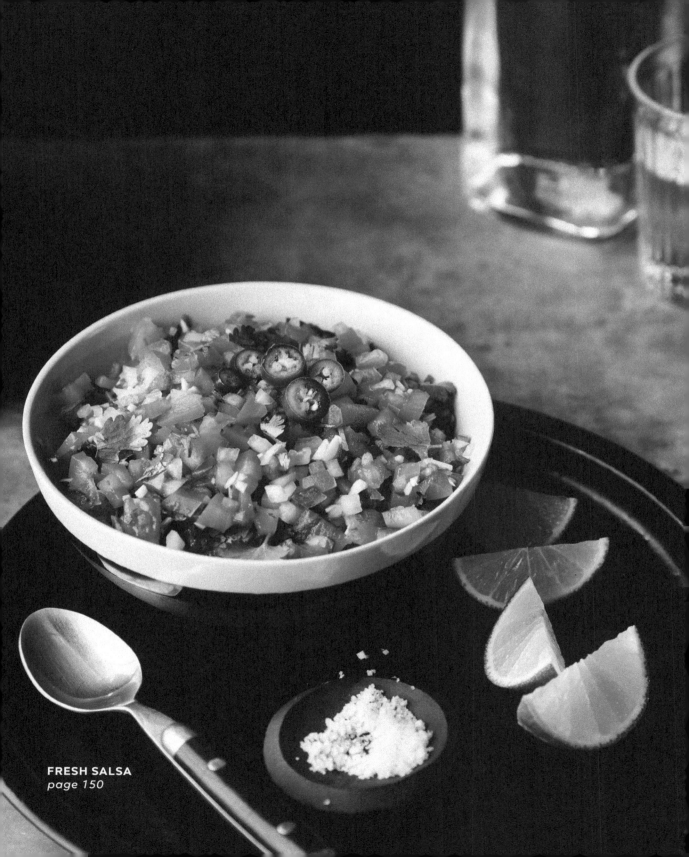

FRESH SALSA
page 150

CHAPTER TEN

KITCHEN STAPLES, CONDIMENTS, AND SAUCES

Fresh Salsa

Yield: 2 cups, Prep time: 10 minutes

30 MINUTES OR LESS, ALLERGEN-FRIENDLY, DAIRY-FREE, NUT-FREE, QUICK PREP, VEGAN/VEGETARIAN

I promise: Once you try this recipe, you'll be hooked on the fresh flavors of this salsa and never buy the jarred stuff again—this is clean eating at its best! Roma tomatoes are my favorite for making salsa, but most varieties will do. If you grow your own vegetables, make this salsa at the season's peak for an extra-special treat.

6 to 8 Roma tomatoes, seeded and roughly chopped

½ large green bell pepper, roughly chopped

1 small yellow onion, roughly chopped

2 cloves garlic

1 small jalapeño pepper, seeded and chopped

Juice of 1 lime

2 teaspoons kosher salt

¼ cup fresh cilantro leaves

1. In a food processor, combine the tomatoes, bell pepper, onion, garlic, jalapeño, lime juice, salt, and cilantro. Pulse a few times to roughly chop.

2. Continue to pulse until the salsa reaches your desired consistency, stopping to scrape down the sides as necessary.

3. Store in an airtight container in the refrigerator for up to 1 week.

VARIATION TIP: This is not an overly spicy salsa, but if you prefer a milder version, eliminate the jalapeño.

PER ¼ CUP: Total calories: 36; Total fat: 0.8g; Saturated fat: 0g; Carbohydrates: 7g; Sodium: 586mg; Fiber: 1.2g; Protein: 1g

Clean Ketchup

Yield: 1¼ cups, Prep time: 10 minutes

ALLERGEN-FRIENDLY, DAIRY-FREE, NUT-FREE, QUICK PREP, VEGETARIAN

One of the first things I did to clean up my family's diet was to start making my own condiments, like salad dressing, mayonnaise, and ketchup. In most cases, we actually preferred the homemade versions, but creating a winning ketchup recipe took a little longer to perfect. I'm happy to say this one is kid- and husband-approved!

¾ cup no-salt-added tomato sauce

3 tablespoons white vinegar

2 tablespoons tomato paste

2 tablespoons honey

1 teaspoon onion powder

½ teaspoon garlic powder

½ teaspoon sea salt

1. In a small bowl, pour in the tomato sauce, vinegar, tomato paste, honey, onion powder, garlic powder, and salt and whisk well.

2. Store in the refrigerator in an airtight container for up to 2 weeks.

COOKING TIP: If desired, process the mixture in a blender or food processor for a silkier, smoother texture.

PER 2 TABLESPOONS: Total calories: 21; Total fat: 0g; Saturated fat: 0g; Carbohydrates: 5.3g; Sodium: 148.5mg; Fiber: 0.5g; Protein: 0.2g

Marinara Sauce

Yield: 4 cups, Prep time: 5 minutes, Cook time: 20 minutes

5 INGREDIENTS OR LESS, 30 MINUTES OR LESS, ALLERGEN-FRIENDLY, DAIRY-FREE, NUT-FREE, ONE-POT, QUICK PREP, VEGETARIAN

Like many jarred sauces and condiments, store-bought marinara often contains hidden sugars and sodium. This quick marinara contains just a few simple ingredients, is super easy to make, and tastes just as good (if not better!) as your soon-to-be-formerly-favorite pre-made sauces. Think about it—it's how the real stuff is made.

1 teaspoon extra-virgin olive oil

2 teaspoons minced garlic

1 (28-ounce) can crushed tomatoes

1½ teaspoons Italian Seasoning Blend (page 164)

½ teaspoon sea salt

1 teaspoon honey

1. In a large pot over medium-high heat, heat the oil. Add the garlic, then cook and stir for about 1 minute.

2. Add the tomatoes, Italian seasoning, salt, and honey. Stir to combine.

3. Bring the sauce to a low boil, cover, and reduce the heat to low. Simmer for 15 minutes.

COOKING TIP: Save time by doubling this recipe and storing the extra sauce in the freezer for future use.

PER ½ CUP: Total calories: 27; Total fat: 0.6g; Saturated fat: 0.1g; Carbohydrates: 4.6g; Sodium: 276.8mg; Fiber: 1g; Protein: 3.6g

Avocado Oil Mayonnaise

Yield: 24 servings (1 tablespoon each), Prep time: 5 minutes

5 INGREDIENTS OR LESS, DAIRY-FREE, NUT-FREE, QUICK PREP

I've been hooked on this homemade mayonnaise for years. It's delicious, but more importantly, it's made with heart-healthy fats rather than processed vegetable oils. I use it in everything, including chicken and tuna salad, salad dressings, and even casseroles.

1¼ cups avocado oil, divided

1 egg

¾ teaspoon sea salt

2 teaspoons freshly squeezed lemon juice

1. In a food processor, combine ¼ cup of oil, egg, and salt. Pulse until combined.

2. While the processor is running, very slowly drizzle in the remaining oil. The mixture will slowly emulsify to become thick and smooth, like the texture of mayonnaise.

3. Add the lemon juice and pulse again to combine.

4. Store in an airtight container in the refrigerator for up to 2 weeks.

SUBSTITUTION TIP: I've had the best results using avocado oil in this recipe, but olive oil can be substituted, if desired. Just be sure to select a light version or the taste may overpower the mayo.

PER SERVING (1 TABLESPOON): Total calories: 111; Total fat: 11.9g; Saturated fat: 1.7g; Carbohydrates: 0g; Sodium: 75.7mg; Fiber: 0g; Protein: 0.3g

Sesame-Ginger Dressing

Yield: ½ cup, Prep time: 10 minutes

30 MINUTES OR LESS, DAIRY-FREE, NUT-FREE, QUICK PREP, VEGAN/VEGETARIAN

If you've never made homemade dressing, let this be the first recipe you try. Those who try it say it is downright drinkable. This scrumptious dressing is naturally sweetened with dates and contains the perfect combination of sesame, ginger, and garlic. Add this take out-reminiscent dressing to all your favorite salads and dishes.

3 large pitted Medjool dates

¼ cup light soy sauce

2 tablespoons rice vinegar

2 tablespoons avocado oil or extra-virgin olive oil

½ tablespoon sesame oil

1 teaspoon minced garlic

1 teaspoon grated fresh ginger

1. Soak the dates in very hot water for 5 minutes, or until soft. Drain and put in a blender or food processor.

2. Add the soy sauce, vinegar, avocado oil, sesame oil, garlic, and ginger and process until the dates are finely ground and the dressing is creamy.

3. Store the dressing in a Mason jar or airtight container for up to 2 weeks.

SUBSTITUTION TIP: Consider using coconut aminos as a replacement in recipes that call for soy sauce. Coconut aminos is made from the sap of coconut blossoms and has a rich, salty flavor similar to soy sauce, but is much lower in sodium. It also contains high levels of amino acids, vitamins B and C, and potassium, and is a great option for those with gluten and/or soy sensitivities.

PER 2 TABLESPOONS: Total calories: 146; Total fat: 8.7g; Saturated fat: 1.2g; Carbohydrates: 16.8g; Sodium: 530.4mg; Fiber: 1.2g; Protein: 1.4g

Creamy Ranch Dressing

Yield: 1¼ cups, Prep time: 5 minutes

5 INGREDIENTS OR LESS, 30 MINUTES OR LESS, DAIRY-FREE, NUT-FREE, QUICK PREP

Classic ranch dressing gets "cleaned up" in this simple recipe, and it's still everything you crave in a ranch dressing. Those bottled, store-bought dressings may be tasty, but they often contain hydrogenated vegetable oils, high-fructose corn syrup, and loads of preservatives. You can feel good about serving this version to your family without sacrificing any flavor.

1 cup Avocado Oil Mayonnaise (page 153)

¼ cup full-fat coconut milk

2 tablespoons red wine vinegar

2 teaspoons Ranch Seasoning Blend (page 164)

1 tablespoon fresh parsley

1. In a food processor, combine the mayonnaise, coconut milk, vinegar, ranch seasoning, and parsley. Blend until smooth and creamy.

2. Refrigerate in a Mason jar or airtight container for up to 2 weeks.

SERVING TIP: This dressing also doubles as a delicious dip for raw veggies.

PER 1 TABLESPOON: Total calories: 94; Total fat: 10g; Saturated fat: 1.8g; Carbohydrates: 0.1g; Sodium: 68mg; Fiber: 0g; Protein: 0.3g

Sweet and Tangy French Dressing

Yield: 1 cup, Prep time: 5 minutes

5 INGREDIENTS OR LESS, 30 MINUTES OR LESS, DAIRY-FREE, NUT-FREE, QUICK PREP, VEGETARIAN

I was prompted to create this recipe for my husband, who loves traditional French dressing. It features a rich tomato flavor and is creamy, sweet, and tangy. It's great for even more than just your salad greens—make your own "Special Burger Sauce" by combining this dressing with Avocado Oil Mayonnaise (page 153) and some Quick Refrigerator Pickles (page 135).

1½ tablespoons tomato paste

¼ cup white vinegar

½ cup extra-virgin olive oil

1½ tablespoons honey

¼ teaspoon sea salt

In a bowl, whisk the tomato paste, vinegar, olive oil, honey, and salt until completely combined and smooth. Alternatively, add the ingredients to a small Mason jar and shake vigorously.

SUBSTITUTION TIP: White wine vinegar or apple cider vinegar can be substituted for the white vinegar.

PER 2 TABLESPOONS: Total calories: 134; Total fat: 13.5g; Saturated fat: 1.8g; Carbohydrates: 3.9g; Sodium: 98.7mg; Fiber: 0.2g; Protein: 0.2g

Stir-Fry Sauce

Yield: 1½ cups, Prep time: 5 minutes

30 MINUTES OR LESS, DAIRY-FREE, ONE-POT, QUICK PREP

The Cashew Chicken Skillet (page 106) and Pork and Broccoli Stir-Fry (page 128) call for this sauce, but it will add robust flavor to any mix of ingredients that you might want to cook in a wok.

⅔ cup light soy sauce

½ cup Basic Homemade Chicken Stock (see Variation tip, page 163)

2 tablespoons rice vinegar

2 tablespoons honey

1 tablespoon arrowroot powder

2 teaspoons sesame oil

1 teaspoon garlic powder

1 teaspoon ginger powder

1 teaspoon cayenne pepper hot sauce (optional)

1. In a Mason jar, combine the soy sauce, stock, rice vinegar, honey, arrowroot powder, sesame oil, garlic powder, ginger powder, and hot sauce (if using). Seal tightly and shake until completely combined.

2. Use immediately or store in the refrigerator for up to 2 weeks.

3. Before using, shake the jar again to mix ingredients.

INGREDIENT TIP: Arrowroot powder is a grain-free alternative to cornstarch that is used as a thickening agent in sauces. You can usually find it in the baking aisle of your grocery store.

PER ½ CUP: Total calories: 140; Total fat: 3g; Saturated fat: 0.4g; Carbohydrates: 26.6g; Sodium: 1,933.5mg; Fiber: 0.2g; Protein: 3.8g

Party Guacamole

Yield: 10 servings, Prep time: 10 minutes

30 MINUTES OR LESS, ALLERGEN-FRIENDLY, DAIRY-FREE, NUT-FREE, ONE-POT, QUICK PREP, VEGAN/VEGETARIAN

Like salsa, fresh guacamole takes advantage of all the vibrance that can only be achieved when you cut up the ingredients yourself. Get creative with its applications, keeping it in mind as an appetizer for parties or a topping for burgers, tacos, eggs, and wraps.

3 large ripe avocados, peeled, pitted, and diced

3 tablespoons freshly squeezed lime juice

2 teaspoons kosher salt

½ teaspoon cumin

3 tablespoons minced red onion

1 Roma tomato, seeded and diced

1 tablespoon chopped fresh cilantro

1. Put the avocados in a medium bowl and mash with a fork.

2. Add the lime juice, salt, and cumin, and mix well.

3. Fold in the red onion, tomato, and cilantro.

4. Store covered, with plastic wrap touching the guacamole, until ready to use. Guacamole is best served within 1 to 2 days—stirring it will freshen up the color again.

INGREDIENT TIP: Find the best avocados by looking for those that have a darker skin and a slight give when pressed with your fingertips. If the avocado feels squishy, it is likely overripe. To ripen an avocado quickly, place in a paper bag with other produce (like bananas). No paper bag? Countertop proximity to other ripening produce will do the trick.

PER SERVING: Total calories: 103; Total fat: 8.8g; Saturated fat: 1.2g; Carbohydrates: 6.1g; Sodium: 470mg; Fiber: 4.4g; Protein: 1.4g

Tzatziki Sauce

Yield: 1 cup, Prep time: 15 minutes

NUT-FREE, QUICK PREP, VEGETARIAN

Tzatziki with its garlicky undertones is delicious paired with meats, salads, and veggies. High in protein from the Greek yogurt, this healthy condiment deserves to be enjoyed often.

¼ **large English cucumber, grated**

¾ **teaspoon sea salt, divided**

¾ **cup plain Greek yogurt**

1 **tablespoon extra-virgin olive oil**

½ **tablespoon red wine vinegar**

1 **teaspoon minced garlic**

1 **tablespoon minced fresh dill**

1. Put the grated cucumber in a fine-mesh strainer, add ¼ teaspoon of salt, and let stand for at least 10 minutes. Lightly press to squeeze out the excess liquid. Set aside.

2. In a bowl, combine the yogurt, olive oil, red wine vinegar, garlic, and remaining salt. Mix well.

3. Fold in the dill and grated cucumber. Cover and chill until ready to serve.

INGREDIENT TIP: Adding salt to the grated cucumber helps release excess moisture so you don't end up with an overly watery sauce.

PER ¼ CUP: Total calories: 86; Total fat: 7.3g; Saturated fat: 2.4g; Carbohydrates: 2.9g; Sodium: 460.7mg; Fiber: 0.1g; Protein: 2.7g

Greek Yogurt Dill Dip

Yield: 1 cup, Prep time: 5 minutes, plus 1 hour resting time

5 INGREDIENTS OR LESS, NUT-FREE, QUICK PREP, VEGETARIAN

It takes no time at all to whip up a savory veggie dip at home. You'll enjoy having this dip on hand with some prepared veggies for an easy snack when the urge for a nosh strikes.

1 cup plain Greek yogurt

2 teaspoons dried dill

1 teaspoon light soy sauce (or coconut aminos)

1 teaspoon sea salt

½ teaspoon garlic powder

½ teaspoon onion powder

1. In a small bowl, combine the yogurt, dill, soy sauce, salt, garlic powder, and onion powder and stir well.

2. Refrigerate for at least 1 hour to let the flavors meld before serving.

3. Store covered in the refrigerator for up to 1 week.

INGREDIENT TIP: Fresh dill can be used in place of dried.

PER ¼ CUP: Total calories: 70; Total fat: 5.5g; Saturated fat: 3.5g; Carbohydrates: 3.5g; Sodium: 80mg; Fiber: 0.1g; Protein: 2.3g

Creamy Hummus

Yield: 2 cups, Prep time: 10 minutes

**5 INGREDIENTS OR LESS, 30 MINUTES OR LESS, QUICK PREP,
VEGAN/VEGETARIAN**

This basic hummus recipe is slightly tangy and super creamy. Get creative with it—serve it with raw veggies, on burgers or wraps, or even in deviled eggs.

2 cups chickpeas, drained and rinsed

¼ cup tahini

¼ cup freshly squeezed lemon juice

2½ tablespoons water, plus more as needed

1 teaspoon minced garlic

1 teaspoon kosher salt

1. In a food processor, combine the chickpeas, tahini, lemon juice, water, garlic, and salt.

2. Process until smooth and creamy. If needed, add more water to reach desired consistency.

VARIATION TIP: Recreate the variety you can find at the supermarket in the comfort of your own home. Try adding some minced garlic and a swirl of olive oil, or a Greek-inspired topping of finely diced olives, cucumbers, and tomatoes. Mix it up!

PER ¼ CUP: Total calories: 114; Total fat: 5.1g; Saturated fat: 0.7g; Carbohydrates: 13.6g; Sodium: 302mg; Fiber: 3.9g; Protein: 5g

All-Purpose Marinades

Prep time: 5 minutes, plus 30 minutes marinating time

ALLERGEN-FRIENDLY, DAIRY-FREE, NUT-FREE, QUICK PREP, VEGETARIAN

All-Purpose Marinades add big flavor to recipes with very little effort, and without all the store-bought version additives. These classic flavor combinations are perfect for grilling, baking, and roasting proteins and vegetables.

For the Rosemary and Dijon Marinade

¼ cup light soy sauce (or coconut aminos)

2 tablespoons extra-virgin olive oil

1½ tablespoons Dijon mustard

2 teaspoons chopped fresh rosemary

1 teaspoon minced garlic

For the Lemon and

Garlic Marinade

½ cup freshly squeezed lemon juice

¼ cup extra-virgin olive oil

1 tablespoon minced garlic

1 teaspoon kosher salt

1 teaspoon honey

½ teaspoon freshly ground black pepper

For the Balsamic and Herbs Marinade

½ cup balsamic vinegar

¼ cup extra-virgin olive oil

2 tablespoons honey

1 tablespoon chopped fresh thyme leaves

1 tablespoon chopped fresh parsley leaves

1 tablespoon kosher salt

1. Combine all the ingredients in a small Mason jar, seal lid, and shake vigorously until combined.

2. Pour over the protein or vegetables, cover, and marinate for at least 30 minutes.

COOKING TIP: To prepare pre-made marinated meats, combine meat and marinade in a large freezer-safe plastic bag, squeeze out the excess air, seal, and freeze until ready to use.

Basic Homemade Broth/Stock

Yield: 10 cups, Prep time: 5 minutes, Cook time: 5 hours

ALLERGEN-FRIENDLY, DAIRY-FREE, NUT-FREE, QUICK PREP, VEGAN/VEGETARIAN

Super clean eating, money-saving, waste-reducing hack: Keep a large resealable freezer bag in your refrigerator or freezer for saving veggie scraps and wilted herbs. When the bag is full, it's time to make broth! See the tip for a Basic Homemade Chicken or Beef Stock variation. Add the optional turmeric for its powerful anti-inflammatory properties.

6 cups (or 1-gallon bag) vegetable scraps from carrots, celery, onions, herbs, etc. (peels, ends, and stems)

10 cups water

2 teaspoons kosher salt

2 bay leaves

1 tablespoon apple cider vinegar

1 teaspoon turmeric powder (optional)

1. Put the vegetable scraps in a slow cooker. Pour the water over the scraps and add the salt, bay leaves, apple cider vinegar, and turmeric (if using). Stir to combine.

2. Cook on high for 5 to 6 hours or on low for 8 to 10 hours.

3. Strain the solids through a fine-mesh sieve. Store the broth in large Mason jars in the refrigerator for up to three days. Broth can also be frozen for up to 3 to 4 months.

VARIATION TIP: To make Basic Homemade Chicken or Beef Stock, add the bones from a whole chicken or cut of beef and reduce the amount of veggie scraps and herbs to 2 cups. Or ask your local butcher for bones for making stock. You can also freeze leftover bones until ready to make.

PER SERVING: Total calories: 10; Total fat: 0g; Saturated fat: 0g; Carbohydrates: 2.5g; Sodium: 465mg; Fiber: 0g; Protein: 0g

Seasoning Blends

Yield: ~7 tablespoons per batch, Prep time: 15 minutes

30 MINUTES OR LESS, ALLERGEN-FRIENDLY, DAIRY-FREE, NUT-FREE, QUICK PREP, VEGAN/VEGETARIAN

Make mealtime easier with these convenient make-ahead seasoning blends using dried ingredients. You'll save time (and money) and always have the perfect flavor booster on hand for your recipes.

For the Cajun Seasoning Blend

2½ tablespoons sea salt

1 tablespoon oregano

1 tablespoon paprika

1 tablespoon cayenne pepper

1 tablespoon freshly ground black pepper

1½ teaspoons garlic powder

1 teaspoon onion powder

For the Chili Seasoning Blend

2½ tablespoons chili powder

1 tablespoon cumin

1 tablespoon paprika or smoked paprika

1 tablespoon onion powder

½ tablespoon oregano

1 teaspoon sea salt

1 teaspoon freshly ground black pepper

For the Mediterranean Seasoning Blend

2 tablespoons basil

2 tablespoons oregano

2 tablespoons kosher salt

1 tablespoon parsley

1 tablespoon dried minced onion

1 teaspoon freshly ground black pepper

For the Italian Seasoning Blend

4 teaspoons basil

4 teaspoons oregano

4 teaspoons rosemary

4 teaspoons marjoram

4 teaspoons thyme

4 teaspoons savory

2 teaspoons garlic powder

For the Ranch Seasoning Blend

2½ tablespoons parsley

2½ teaspoons garlic powder

2½ teaspoons onion powder

2 teaspoons dried dill

2 teaspoons dried minced onion

1½ teaspoons sea salt

1 teaspoon freshly ground black pepper

For the Poultry Seasoning Blend

2 tablespoons ground sage

1½ tablespoons thyme

1 tablespoon marjoram

1 tablespoon rosemary

½ tablespoon nutmeg

½ tablespoon freshly ground black pepper

For the Taco and Fajita Seasoning Blend

2 tablespoons chili powder

4 teaspoons cumin

2 teaspoons coriander

2 teaspoons sea salt

1 teaspoon onion powder

1 teaspoon garlic powder

1 teaspoon oregano

1 teaspoon smoked paprika

½ teaspoon freshly ground black pepper

¼ teaspoon chipotle powder (optional)

1. In a small bowl, combine the ingredients for the desired seasoning blend. Stir well to combine. Pour into individual Mason jars or airtight containers.

2. Before using, stir the seasoning blends well, as spices can tend to settle.

3. Spices using dried ingredients can be stored for several months.

VARIATION TIP: Feel free to reduce the salt content in any of these recipes if you are concerned about your sodium intake.

MEASUREMENT CONVERSIONS

Volume Equivalents (Liquid)

US STANDARD	US STANDARD (OUNCES)	METRIC (APPROXIMATE)
2 tablespoons	1 fl. oz.	30 mL
¼ cup	2 fl. oz.	60 mL
½ cup	4 fl. oz.	120 mL
1 cup	8 fl. oz.	240 mL
1½ cups	12 fl. oz.	355 mL
2 cups or 1 pint	16 fl. oz.	475 mL
4 cups or 1 quart	32 fl. oz.	1 L
1 gallon	128 fl. oz.	4 L

Oven Temperatures

FAHRENHEIT (F)	CELSIUS (C) (APPROXIMATE)
250°F	120°C
300°F	150°C
325°F	165°C
350°F	180°C
375°F	190°C
400°F	200°C
425°F	220°C
450°F	230°C

Volume Equivalents (Dry)

US STANDARD	METRIC (APPROXIMATE)
⅛ teaspoon	0.5 mL
¼ teaspoon	1 mL
½ teaspoon	2 mL
¾ teaspoon	4 mL
1 teaspoon	5 mL
1 tablespoon	15 mL
¼ cup	59 mL
⅓ cup	79 mL
½ cup	118 mL
⅔ cup	156 mL
¾ cup	177 mL
1 cup	235 mL
2 cups or 1 pint	475 mL
3 cups	700 mL
4 cups or 1 quart	1 L

Weight Equivalents

US STANDARD	METRIC (APPROXIMATE)
½ ounce	15 g
1 ounce	30 g
2 ounces	60 g
4 ounces	115 g
8 ounces	225 g
12 ounces	340 g
16 ounces or 1 pound	455 g

RESOURCES

Clean Eating Books

In Defense of Food by Michael Pollan

Food Rules: An Eater's Manual by Michael Pollan

The Primal Blueprint by Mark Sisson

*Food Can Fix It: The Superfood Switch to Fight Fat,
   Defy Aging, and Eat Your Way Healthy* by Dr. Mehmet Oz

Health, Wellness, and Recipe Websites

Draxe.com

EatingWell.com

EatWellGuide.org

EWG.org/FoodScore

Prevention.com

RobbWolf.com

Tastythin.com

ThePaleoMom.com

Whole30.com

YogaWithAdriene.com

Health and Wellness Podcasts

The Paleo Solution by Robb Wolf

The Wellness Mama by Katie Wells

Balanced Bites by Diane Sanfilippo

Bulletproof Radio by Dave Asprey

Fitness, Nutrition, and Exercise Apps

MyFitnessPal

Pocket Yoga

MyFitness by Jillian Michaels

8Fit

Couch to 5K

REFERENCES

Ballantyne, Sarah. *Paleo Principles*. Tuttle Publishing, 2017.

Haas, Elson M., and Buck Levin. *Staying Healthy with Nutrition: The Complete Guide to Diet and Nutritional Medicine*. Celestial Arts, 2006.

Glassman, Keri. "Kale: The Leafy Green Full of Vitamins." WebMD. Accessed December 16, 2019. webmd.com/food-recipes/features/why-is-kale-good-for-me#1.

"Study Suggests Home Cooking Is a Main Ingredient in Healthier Diet—Johns Hopkins Center for a Livable Future." *Center for a Livable Future*. November 17, 2014. clf.jhsph.edu/about-us/news/news-2014/study-suggests-home-cooking-main-ingredient-healthier-diet.

"How Are Food and the Environment Related?" *Taking Charge of Your Health & Wellbeing*. 2016. takingcharge.csh.umn.edu/explore-healing-practices/food-medicine/how-are-food-and-environment-related.

Kovacs, Jenny Stamos. "The Dos and Don'ts of Counting Calories." WebMD. 2009. webmd.com/diet/features/dos-donts-counting-calories#3.

Cheryl, Fryar D, et al. "Products - Health E Stats - Overweight, Obesity, and Extreme Obesity Among Adults 2011–2012." Centers for Disease Control and Prevention. September 2014. cdc.gov/nchs/data/hestat/obesity_adult_11_12/obesity_adult_11_12.htm.

"Why Good Nutrition Is Important." *Center for Science in the Public Interest*. Accessed December 16, 2019. cspinet.org/eating-healthy/why-good-nutrition-important.

Steele, Euridice Martínez, et al. "The Share of Ultra-Processed Foods and the Overall Nutritional Quality of Diets in the US: Evidence from a Nationally Representative Cross-Sectional Study." *Population Health Metrics* 15, no. 1 (2017). doi.org/10.1186/s12963-017-0119-3.

"Fruit and Vegetables." *Linus Pauling Institute*: Micronutrient Information Center. Accessed October 22, 2019. lpi.oregonstate.edu/mic/food-beverages /fruit-vegetables.

INDEX

C

ACKNOWLEDGMENTS

First of all, to my husband, John, who never once doubted me all those years ago when I had the crazy idea to start a blog—thank you for your unwavering support and faith in everything I do.

Thank you to my family, friends, and supporters for being my cheerleaders on this journey. Especially to Avery and Keira, my biggest fans—you are my inspiration and greatest accomplishment in life. A special thank-you goes to my parents, and to my grandma Ann who knew how to express her love through food and is always with me in spirit.

To say I am honored and thrilled to be writing this book is an understatement. It is a dream come true that I will be forever grateful for.

ABOUT THE AUTHOR

 NIKKI BEHNKE is a nutritional therapy student, blogger, and writer. A graduate of the University of Michigan, she is the owner and creator of the website Tastythin.com, where she develops and shares real food, family-friendly recipes, and meal plans. Studying nutrition and inspiring others to live a clean-eating lifestyle is her greatest passion. She lives in Michigan with her husband, two daughters, and dog, Rosie.

CPSIA information can be obtained
at www.ICGtesting.com
Printed in the USA
JSHW012112280220
4448JS00001B/1